Glossary

Achalasia: a condition in which the normal muscular activity of the oesophagus is disturbed, delaying the passage of swallowed material

Achlorhydria: absence of free hydrochloric acid in the stomach

Barrett's epithelium: columnar cell lining of the oesophagus instead of normal squamous cells, induced by chronic acid reflux. It is associated with an increased incidence of cancer

CLO test: test for *Campylobacter*-like organism, the old description of *H. pylori* before it was reclassified

Dysphagia: a condition in which the action of swallowing is difficult to perform or in which swallowed material seems to be held up in its passage to the stomach

EGG: electrogastrogram, a recording of the myoelectrical rhythm of the stomach

Eradication treatment: pharmacological therapy that aims to eradicate *H. pylori* from the stomach. Most commonly used regimens comprise a proton-pump inhibitor and two antibiotics, given over 7 days

Gastroparesis: paralysis of the stomach resulting in delayed gastric emptying

GORD/GERD: gastro-oesophageal reflux disease (GERD is the US term)

LOS/LES: lower oesophageal sphincter (LES is the US term); normal LOS pressure is 22 ± 8 mmHg

MALT: mucosa-associated lymphoid tissue

Meckel's diverticulum: a pouch in the wall of the distal ileum; it is a congenital abnormality

Nissen fundoplication: the most commonly performed surgical procedure for GORD; the gastric fundus is wrapped around itself and the distal oesophagus and any hiatal hernia is reduced

Odynophagia: pain on swallowing, rather than a burning sensation rising into the retrosternal area

Oesophagitis: inflammation of the oesophagus usually due to excessive exposure to refluxed gastric acid

Torsades de pointes: tachycardia in which the electrical stimulation of the heart undergoes a cyclical variation in strength; it gives a characteristic pattern of twisted spikes on the electrocardiogram

UBT: urea breath test, a non-invasive test for establishing current *H. pylori* infection

UGI: upper gastrointestinal

Zollinger-Ellison syndrome: condition characterized by excess production of gastrin usually due to a G cell tumour of the pancreas; this leads to hypersecretion of gastric acid and ulceration of the oesophagus, stomach, duodenum and jejunum

Introduction

The term 'dyspepsia' defies precise definition, but is generally understood to mean symptoms suggestive of upper gastrointestinal (UGI) disease (Table 1). Dyspepsia may be caused by many conditions, including diseases of the pancreas and biliary system, but the majority of patients with dyspepsia have an organic or functional disorder of the upper alimentary tract (Table 2).

Dyspepsia is extremely common in western society, with a prevalence of 25–40% over a 6–12-month period. Only 25% of sufferers consult a doctor; they do so not only as a result of symptom severity, but also because of concern about potentially sinister disease.

Although dyspepsia accounts for approximately 5% of family physician consultations in the USA and UK, only a fraction of patients are referred to specialists. In the UK, for example, only about 10% of patients with dyspepsia are referred for specialist investigation. Despite this, 2% of the UK population now annually undergo UGI endoscopy or barium-meal examination.

The economic consequences of dyspepsia are impressive. In the UK, nearly 9 million prescriptions were written for H_2-receptor antagonists in 1993. In the same year, over £400 million was spent on ulcer-healing drugs. In addition, sales of over-the-counter antacids accounted for £65 million. Worldwide expenditure on ulcer drugs for 1998 was approximately US$11 000 million; US$4000 million were spent on proton-pump inhibitors alone, of which nearly 50% were consumed in the USA.

TABLE 1

Symptoms of dyspepsia

• Upper abdominal pain/discomfort	• Regurgitation
• Anorexia	• Bloating
• Belching	• Early satiety
• Heartburn	• Nausea and/or vomiting

TABLE 2

Definitions of dyspepsia

Organic dyspepsia

Symptoms due to specific abnormalities, either:

- morphological (peptic ulcer, gastro-oesophageal carcinoma and oesophagitis detected by UGI endoscopy), or

- pathophysiological (gastro-oesophageal reflux, detected by pH monitoring; gastroparesis, detected by solid-phase gastric-emptying tests)

Functional dyspepsia: ulcer-like and dysmotility-like functional dyspepsia

Symptoms for which mechanisms have been proposed, but are poorly understood and for which confirmatory investigations are not generally available (delayed gastric emptying and other gut-motility or sensitivity disorders)

Non-ulcer dyspepsia

In the past, this has meant ulcer-like symptoms in the absence of proven ulcer. Strictly it ought to include all causes of dyspepsia not due to peptic ulcer. Recently it has been used synonymously with ulcer-like dyspepsia. Non-ulcer dyspepsia is a confusing term and ideally should be discarded

Indirect costs and social consequences of dyspepsia are more difficult to measure. A UK survey in 1994 revealed that 40% of those with gastro-oesophageal reflux, 46% of gastric ulcer sufferers and 59% of duodenal ulcer patients had lost time from work in the previous 12 months due to their disease.

Fast Facts – Dyspepsia provides an up-to-date account of our understanding of the main causes of dyspepsia and their management in the context of general practice.

CHAPTER 1

Approaching uninvestigated dyspepsia

Patients with dyspepsia are not a homogeneous group and therefore selection and prioritization are required.

Patients not requiring immediate investigation

Patients under the age of 45 years with a short history of dyspepsia may be treated empirically for 4–6 weeks, in the absence of alarm symptoms (Table 1.1). This approach prevents unnecessary investigation of many young patients with so-called 'self-limiting' dyspepsia and supposedly reduces management costs and inconvenience. Such a policy is valid providing:
- a significant proportion of young dyspeptics fall into this category
- the majority do not return because symptoms resolve or are subsequently controlled by over-the-counter drugs and lifestyle changes.

The overall success of this approach depends on:
- appropriate selection of patients
- the physician's clinical diagnostic skills
- the physician's ability to reassure and convince the patient that immediate investigation is unnecessary.

If not applied appropriately, however, the 'treat-before-investigation' approach may delay optimal management and prove less cost-effective.

Symptom clusters. It has been proposed that clusters of symptoms might be used as a guide to initial therapy of dyspepsia in young, uninvestigated patients (Table 1.2).

TABLE 1.1

Alarm symptoms

- Anaemia
- Bleeding
- Dysphagia
- Persistent vomiting
- Weight loss/anorexia

7

TABLE 1.2

Symptom clusters in uninvestigated dyspepsia

Gastro-oesophageal reflux disease-like

- Heartburn
- Regurgitation

Ulcer-like

- Localized epigastric pain
- Nocturnal pain
- Relief with antacids or vomiting

Dysmotility-like

- Poorly localized pain or discomfort
- Early satiety
- Bloating
- Nausea

- Dyspepsia symptoms, like those associated with gastro-oesophageal reflux disease (GORD, or GERD in the USA), may be treated with an alginate/antacid if symptoms are mild. If symptoms are more severe and unresponsive, prokinetic or anti-secretory drugs should be prescribed.
- When ulcer-like dyspepsia is suspected, an H_2-receptor antagonist would be an appropriate initial choice.
- If dysmotility symptoms predominate, a prokinetic agent should be taken in the first instance.

This approach to early management is advocated on the assumption that, in each of these categories, the implied pathogenesis is operative in a substantial number of patients and that drug therapy selected on this basis has a reasonable chance of being effective. Unfortunately, many patients do not fall neatly into one particular category, which reduces the therapeutic potential of the classification. Furthermore, it must be emphasized that this is a clinical classification and that the implied pathogenesis is not proved. Therefore, if an apparently logical first-choice therapy is ineffective after

2–3 weeks, an alternative class of drug should be prescribed. If this fails, investigation or referral should follow without delay.

Helicobacter pylori **serological screening.** Because of the close association between *H. pylori* and organic causes of dyspepsia, serological screening has been used to guide initial management of young patients. One proposal is that *H. pylori*-positive patients should be referred for endoscopy and given eradication treatment if ulcer disease is confirmed. In the UK, this approach is probably not appropriate in general practice.

The alternative policy is to treat all young, *H. pylori*-positive dyspeptics without alarm features (see Table 1.1) with eradication therapy. The rationale is that 25% will have ulcers, many others will have relevant responsive mucosal lesions and for the remainder, there is the potential to reduce the risk of future disease. This approach is advocated by the Primary Care Group of the British Society of Gastroenterology and is supported by prospective studies. However, the personal approach of one of the authors, Kenneth Koch, is to treat only documented ulcers in patients with dyspepsia and positive *H. pylori* tests.

H. pylori-negative patients in this age group are unlikely to have major organic disease. Therefore, they may be treated symptomatically and only referred if unresponsive.

Patients requiring early investigation or referral

Patients with alarm features. Regardless of their age, all patients who have one or more alarm symptom (Table 1.1) should be investigated promptly. These symptoms are frequently associated with serious organic disease.

Patients over 45 years of age. The risk of organic disease increases with age. Any patient over 45 with recent onset of dyspepsia should be referred or investigated without delay, regardless of *H. pylori* status.

Patients with chronic symptoms. Many previously uninvestigated patients with significant long-standing dyspeptic symptoms will have chronic organic disease. Those who have used antacids in large quantities on an almost daily basis for several years are particularly likely to have peptic disease. They need to be distinguished from those with non-acid-related functional dyspepsia to optimize future management.

Anxious or phobic patients. Some patients or their relatives will be dissatisfied with a clinically based diagnosis. Early referral should then be conceded to facilitate future management. These patients include those with:

- excessive anxiety
- cancer phobia
- a vulnerable psychosocial background
- an associate with a recent history of serious disease.

Initial investigations

Upper gastrointestinal endoscopy is undoubtedly the most appropriate initial investigation, because of its capacity to confirm or exclude the majority of diseases that commonly cause dyspepsia (Table 1.3). The procedure is highly cost-effective because it often reduces the need for subsequent consultations and helps the physician to optimize drug therapy. As a result, most gastroenterologists strongly believe that patients with persistent or recurrent dyspepsia should undergo this investigation.

TABLE 1.3

Endoscopy can identify conditions often associated with dyspepsia*

Finding	Patients (%)
Normal	38.0
Peptic ulcer	18.0
Oesophagitis	15.0
Gastritis	18.0
Duodenitis	8.0
Carcinoma	1.8
Miscellaneous	1.2

*Data from Jones 1989

Abdominal ultrasound scanning has very limited value in the routine investigation of dyspepsia and should be reserved for patients with suspected biliary colic, cholecystitis, bile-duct obstruction or pancreatic disease. Note that vague pain in the right hypochondrium and flatulence, once thought to be symptoms of cholelithiasis, are no more common in patients with gallstones than in those without.

Biochemical tests. Confirmed anaemia increases the suspicion that dyspepsia has an organic cause. Abnormal liver biochemistry is found in some patients with biliary tract and pancreatic disease. However, the majority of dyspeptic patients have normal blood tests.

CHAPTER 2
Gastro-oesophageal reflux disease

Symptoms of GORD often result from disordered oesophagogastric motility, which facilitates the escape of normally secreted gastric acid into the distal oesophagus for an abnormally long time.

Pathophysiology

The pathophysiology of GORD encompasses a continuum ranging from:

- reflux of small amounts of acid with persistent symptoms, to
- severe ulceration with stricture formation and dysphagia, to
- an inflammatory alteration of mucosal epithelium, to
- intestinal dysplasia, cellular atypia and adenocarcinoma.

Small amounts of acid reflux from the stomach into the oesophagus occur on a daily basis in healthy individuals. Studies indicate that, for 1–6% of a 24-hour day, pH in the distal oesophagus transiently falls below 4. So, for most of the time, acid in the stomach lumen is retained in the stomach.

Normal neuromuscular activities of the oesophagus and stomach (oesophagogastric motility) ensure that acid remains in the stomach or is emptied into the duodenum, and that very little refluxes into the oesophagus. These activities include:

- normal oesophageal peristalsis
- normal lower oesophageal sphincter (LOS) pressure
- a normal number of transient LOS relaxations
- normal gastric emptying.

Disorders of oesophageal and gastric motility associated with acidic reflux are listed in Table 2.1. Other oesophageal defences are the cardiac glands within the distal oesophageal squamous epithelium, which secrete bicarbonate, and normal secretion of saliva, which is rich in bicarbonate.

Hypersecretory states present an additional challenge for the neuromuscular and epithelial defences of the oesophagus. In Zollinger-Ellison syndrome, gastric and duodenal ulcerations are the major problems, but 40–60% of patients also have reflux oesophagitis. The majority of

TABLE 2.1

Pathogenesis of GORD

Dysmotility	Toxic refluxates
• Failed oesophageal peristalsis	• Gastric acid
• Decreased amplitude of oesophageal contractions	• Pepsin
	• Bile
• Hypotensive LOS pressure	
• Transient relaxation of LOS pressure	

LOS, lower oesophageal sphincter

patients with GORD, however, have normal acid secretory status and only a minority have idiopathic acid hypersecretion.

Dysfunction of the oesophageal body. Studies from otherwise healthy individuals with GORD have shown that increasing mucosal damage (i.e. from mild to severe oesophagitis) is associated with increasing contractile abnormalities of the oesophageal body. Healthy control subjects fail to elicit a normal oesophageal peristaltic wave after only 10% of voluntary swallows, but patients with severe oesophagitis fail to have normal peristaltic contractions after 30% of voluntary swallows. Thus, swallowed saliva often fails to reach the distal portions of the oesophagus and neutralize refluxed acid (Figure 2.1).

The amplitude of oesophageal contractions may also be decreased in patients with reflux oesophagitis. Even when acute inflammation is healed, neither the amplitude of contractions nor the frequency of normal oesophageal peristalsis improves. Thus, the patient with GORD and oesophagitis has fixed, underlying, oesophageal motility abnormalities.

Dysfunction of the lower oesophageal sphincter. Lower oesophageal sphincter pressure was at one time believed to be the chief defence against GORD (Figure 2.1). Numerous studies showed that patients with severe erosive oesophagitis and regurgitation often had LOS pressures below 10 mmHg (normal LOS pressure is 22 ± 8 mmHg). When LOS pressure is

13

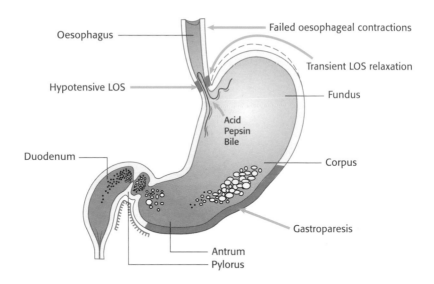

Figure 2.1 Pathophysiology of GORD includes oesophageal and gastric motility disturbances related to failed oesophageal peristalsis, hypotensive lower oesophageal sphincter (LOS), transient and inappropriate relaxation of the LOS, and gastric dysmotility (gastroparesis). Dysmotility allows the reflux of toxic substances (acid, pepsin or bile) into the oesophagus.

below 10 mmHg, small increases in intra-abdominal pressure (such as those that occur when bending over or after eating a large meal) often result in free reflux of gastric content into the oesophagus.

However, many patients with severe heartburn have entirely normal resting LOS pressures. The most common mechanism by which acid refluxes from the stomach into the oesophagus is related to transient and inappropriate LOS relaxations (Figure 2.2). In these instances, the normal resting LOS pressure spontaneously reduces. This transient relaxation presents an opportunity for acid reflux to occur. In mild GORD, there are increased numbers of transient LOS relaxations; as the number of transient relaxations increases, the severity of oesophagitis increases.

Gastric dysmotility. Gastric emptying of chyme occurs, almost linearly, over 90–120 minutes after ingestion of solid foods. Abnormalities in gastric emptying have been recorded in 30–40% of patients with GORD. In some, emptying of standard meals (usually technetium-labelled eggs or liver) is significantly delayed (gastroparesis) compared with control subjects. As gastric acid and chyme remain in the stomach for longer if gastroparesis is present, risk of reflux is increased, particularly when LOS pressure is very low and during transient oesophageal sphincter relaxations.

Gastric acid, bile and pancreatic juices. The most injurious agent in GORD appears to be gastric acid. Most patients with GORD, however, have normal acid secretion. Therefore, normal amounts of acid can cause symptoms and mucosal damage if the oesophageal epithelium is in contact with acid for prolonged periods of time. A small percentage of patients with GORD also reflux bile, with or without acid, into the oesophagus. Pancreatic juices may also be toxic to the squamous epithelium of the distal oesophagus; very little is known about this mechanism of injury.

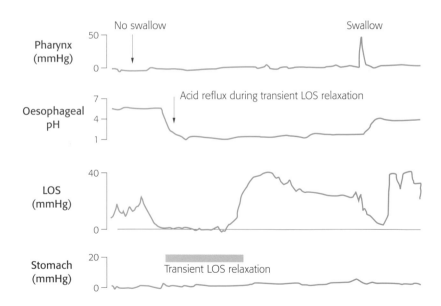

Figure 2.2 Transient LOS relaxation and GORD. In the absence of a swallow, the LOS relaxes to intragastric pressure for a prolonged period of time. After several seconds of transient LOS relaxation, acid reflux occurs as indicated by the decrease in oesophageal pH from 6 to 1. Reproduced with permission from Holloway RH. *Am J Physiol* 1995; 268:G128–33.

Causes of neuromuscular damage to the oesophagus and stomach in most patients with GORD are unknown. However, certain systemic disorders may affect oesophageal neuromuscular function and increase the risk of gastro-oesophageal reflux. With scleroderma, for example, type I collagen is deposited into the submucosal tissues. Eventually, enteric neurones are destroyed and normal smooth muscle cells are replaced with collagen, resulting in decreased oesophageal muscle function. Thus, the amplitude of peristaltic contractions decreases in the oesophageal body until eventually few or no contractions occur in the rigid sclerodermatous oesophageal body. Similarly, LOS pressure decreases markedly in scleroderma as sphincter muscles are weakened and replaced by collagen deposits, and free reflux occurs. Patients with scleroderma and the CRST syndrome (calcinosis, Raynaud's phenomenon, sclerodactyly and telangiectasia), in particular, are at high risk for oesophagitis and oesophagitis-related peptic strictures.

Chronic sequelae. Many patients with chronic reflux and classic heartburn symptoms will have virtually no observable damage in the oesophageal mucosa at endoscopy. Increased eosinophilia and acute inflammatory cells may be seen in histological sections of biopsies from apparently normal distal oesophagus. On the other hand, recurrent acid reflux may lead to obvious oesophageal ulcers.

Oesophagitis is graded from 1 (mild) to 3 (erosive). The intermittent inflammation and healing process may lead to peptic strictures in the distal oesophagus in some patients. Other patients with chronic GORD may develop Barrett's epithelium, which may range from the gastric to the intestinal type. The intestinal type is more likely to develop areas of dysplasia, cellular atypia and adenocarcinoma. Severe atypia is associated with a high risk of adenocarcinoma of the oesophagus.

Symptoms

Diagnosis is based on clinical symptoms, the most common being heartburn (Table 2.2). Atypical GORD symptoms caused by acid reflux into the oesophagus, pharynx, lungs and throat are another important clinical area for consideration. Typical or atypical angina-like chest discomfort, nocturnal asthma attacks, aspiration pneumonia, chronic hoarseness and a variety of other symptoms may be related to gastro-oesophageal reflux.

TABLE 2.2

Clinical symptoms of GORD

Typical

- Heartburn
- Regurgitation
- Belching

Atypical

- Halitosis
- Dental erosions

} May be noted by dentist

- Hoarseness
- Chronic cough

} May be noted by otolaryngologist

- Episodic asthma   May be noted by chest physician

- Substernal discomfort,   May be noted by cardiologist
  angina pectoris

- Nausea
- Early satiety, fullness, bloating
  (associated with gastric dysmotility)

} May be noted by gastroenterologist

Heartburn is the most common symptom associated with GORD. It is defined as a burning sensation high in the epigastrium that *rises* into the subxiphoid or substernal areas. Burning may be felt higher in the retrosternal region and into the back of the throat. Heartburn may be accompanied by increased salivation or pressure discomfort in the retrosternal area. It typically occurs in the postprandial hours and may also occur at night when the patient is supine. Nocturnal heartburn is associated with increased severity of oesophagitis and stricture formation.

In most people, heartburn is transient and related to over-indulgence of a wide variety of rich or acidic foods. Over-the-counter antacids have traditionally been the treatment of choice for simple heartburn. The recently available over-the-counter H_2-receptor antagonists have given individuals access to systemic medications to decrease gastric-acid secretion and reduce self-diagnosed heartburn symptoms. However, millions of patients have persistent and chronic heartburn symptoms that are troublesome and may also lead to serious sequelae, such as:

- gastrointestinal bleeding from oesophageal erosions and ulcers
- peptic stricture formation
- formation of Barrett's epithelium, with an attendant increase in the incidence of adenocarcinoma of the oesophagus.

Alarm symptoms. If the patient is over 50 years of age and has heartburn and one or more alarm symptoms (Table 2.3), heartburn should be addressed with more aggressive diagnostic and therapeutic action.

Dysphagia for solids, but not liquids, may indicate mechanical obstruction of the oesophagus. The key possibilities include:

- peptic stricture
- oesophageal rings or webs
- distal oesophageal squamous cell carcinoma or adenocarcinoma.

Odynophagia (pain on swallowing, rather than a burning sensation rising into the retrosternal area) suggests an infectious oesophagitis caused by *Candida* or herpes simplex virus. Immunocompromised patients may have one of these atypical causes of their heartburn or odynophagia. Weight loss, melaena or anaemia suggest the possibility of oesophageal or gastric cancer. Scleroderma and pill-induced oesophagitis should be considered. Potassium tablets, salicylates and foscarnet are frequent causes of pill-induced oesophagitis.

Atypical symptoms. Over the past several years, interest in atypical presentations of GORD has increased from medical and surgical specialties, ranging from dentistry to cardiology (see Table 2.2). Atypical symptoms

TABLE 2.3

Alarm symptoms

- Dysphagia
- Odynophagia
- Weight loss
- Blood in regurgitant fluids or vomitus

that may present in the dental realm include loss of dental enamel and halitosis. Ear, nose and throat physicians have determined that patients with chronic hoarseness and sore throat frequently have occult GORD. Many of these patients do not report heartburn symptoms. If present, they may be unimportant to the patient compared with the throat symptoms.

Pulmonary physicians appreciate that gastro-oesophageal reflux is frequently present in asthmatic patients. Nocturnal asthma attacks or microaspiration may be precipitated by GORD. Similarly, chronic cough is stimulated by gastro-oesophageal reflux in some patients. In a recent study, patients with severe chronic obstructive pulmonary or bronchospastic disease underwent Nissen fundoplication (see pages 24–25); the incidence of reflux and severity of pulmonary symptoms decreased significantly as a result.

In other patients, reflux of acid into the oesophagus is perceived as a pressure discomfort or heaviness rather than a burning sensation. Some patients may have no burning at all and acid reflux is experienced as a squeezing pressure or substernal pain that suggests angina pectoris. Reflux of acid into the oesophagus probably causes an angina-like pain by either:
- stimulating a sensory reflex
- inducing focal ischaemia in the oesophageal muscular wall
- stimulating oesophageal smooth muscle spasm.

Other gastrointestinal symptoms may be associated with GORD. In a series of patients with chronic unexplained nausea, occult GORD was present and episodes of nausea were associated with acid reflux recorded during 24-hour oesophageal pH studies. Aggressive anti-secretory and promotility therapy improved the nausea.

Many patients with heartburn also have symptoms associated with gastric emptying disorders, such as excess postprandial fullness, early satiety and epigastric discomfort. These patients have an overlap syndrome in which GORD and symptoms associated with gastroparesis are present.

Finally, patients with Barrett's epithelium may have very minor heartburn symptoms. As the squamous mucosa changes to the gastric or intestinal type, it becomes less sensitive to acid exposure from a symptomatic view-point. In patients who have had mild reflux for many years, the possibility of Barrett's epithelium should be considered.

Diagnosis

The basic approach to the management of GORD is to make the clinical diagnosis in patients with classical symptoms and to be suspicious of GORD in patients with atypical symptoms. In the patient with classical symptoms of GORD, it is important to consider underlying systemic disorders that might be causing the symptoms and to check for the presence of alarm symptoms as described previously. The presence of dysphagia and the chronicity of relatively mild heartburn should also raise concerns regarding Barrett's epithelium and the complications thereof. Dysphagia, odynophagia or other alarm symptoms indicate that a more aggressive and definitive diagnostic approach should be taken.

Barium-swallow examination is the minimum oesophageal evaluation required for patients with one or more alarm symptom. Barium-swallow radiographs will show large ulcers, masses and other structural defects that may be causing the symptoms. Structural defects detected on barium swallow must be evaluated with UGI endoscopy and be biopsied for malignancy if suspicious. Depending on the services available, UGI endoscopy should be the initial diagnostic procedure of choice in the presence of alarm symptoms.

Endoscopy. As the intensity of heartburn symptoms does not correlate well with endoscopic findings, it is helpful to use endoscopy for those patients who have classical GORD symptoms but are not responding to standard treatment approaches (see page 21). Upper endoscopic examination may reveal an entirely normal oesophageal mucosa or a continuum of endoscopic findings, from streaky erythematous areas to obvious ulcerations of the squamous epithelium. Peptic or cancerous strictures or Barrett's epithelium may be detected. Retained food in the stomach suggests neuromuscular abnormalities of the stomach and large amounts of bile suggest duodenogastric reflux. A solid-phase gastric-emptying study will confirm the diagnosis of gastroparesis. Electrogastrography will indicate the presence of gastric dysrhythmia. These two non-invasive tests of gastric motility are described further in Chapter 6.

Other tests. If barium-swallow or endoscopic studies of the oesophagus, stomach and duodenum are entirely normal and the patient continues to have heartburn despite standard therapies, determination of oesophageal motility and 24-hour pH measurements may be needed. Oesophageal manometry will detect a hypotensive LOS and indicate the continuing high risk for recurrent reflux or regurgitation. On the other hand, the LOS pressure may be normal, which suggests that the main mechanism of reflux is transient relaxation of the sphincter. Other unsuspected oesophageal motility disorders may be found, such as achalasia or findings suggestive of scleroderma. A 24-hour oesophageal pH study will determine the extent to which the oesophageal mucosa is exposed to gastric acid. The patient records all heartburn episodes and the time of symptoms in a diary, so that the physician can correlate reflux events with the occurrence of symptoms. GORD may not, in fact, be documented. A positive result may confirm the diagnosis of GORD as a cause of atypical symptoms.

Atypical GORD symptoms, such as chronic cough, hoarseness, episodic asthma and angina-like chest discomfort require a confirmatory 24-hour oesophageal pH study. The time of symptom occurrence and the correlation between symptoms and individual reflux events should be documented carefully.

Treatment

Treatment of GORD is organized into a series of stages.
- Stage I involves lifestyle and behaviour modifications.
- Stage II consists of treatment with systemic drugs, such as H_2-receptor antagonists, prokinetic agents and proton-pump inhibitors.
- Stage III includes surgical procedures, such as Nissen fundoplication.

Stage I. During this stage, the physician seeks to identify risk factors in the patient's lifestyle that might contribute to GORD symptoms. Certain foods, particularly citric juices, and tomato- and onion-based spices or foods, are commonly associated with increased heartburn symptoms. Chocolate, alcohol and nicotine decrease LOS pressure to some degree and increase the likelihood of reflux symptoms. Other lifestyle changes include decreasing the volume of food ingested at the evening meal and eating at an earlier time to avoid sleeping with a full stomach. The head of the patient's bed may be placed on 4–6 inch (10–15 cm) blocks so that gravity helps to prevent stomach contents from refluxing into the oesophagus.

The physician should also review the patient's medications to identify those drugs that decrease LOS pressure (calcium-channel blockers and drugs containing theophylline) or decrease gastric emptying rates (anticholinergic drugs and opioids). If possible, these drugs should be stopped to see if symptoms improve.

Most patients will have tried over-the-counter antacids. The availability of over-the-counter H_2-receptor antagonists has increased the likelihood that the patient will have tried these drugs; if they do not relieve the symptoms of GORD, patients are often motivated to seek medical attention. Physicians who diagnose GORD typically prescribe H_2-receptor antagonists at higher doses than are available over the counter. Alternatively, prokinetic agents may be prescribed. When stage I approaches fail to relieve symptoms, stage II therapies should be considered.

Stage II. In the presence of classical heartburn symptoms, the physician can address either the acid secretion or the relevant oesophagogastric dysmotility aspects of GORD. H_2-receptor antagonists include cimetidine, ranitidine, nizatidine and famotidine (Table 2.4). They differ in potency, but overall effectiveness is approximately the same. H_2-receptor antagonists heal endoscopically proven oesophagitis in about 50% of patients at 8 weeks and up to 70% at 12 weeks.

Metoclopramide is a centrally and peripherally acting dopamine-2 (D_2) antagonist that increases the LOS pressure and the rate of gastric emptying. It can be given orally or by intravenous infusion. The usual dose is 10 mg, three or four times a day in the UK. In the USA, the usual dose is 10–15 mg, four times a day. However, approximately 20–30% of patients will experience side-effects related to central nervous system events, including depression, anxiety and tardive dyskinesia.

Domperidone is a drug with a similar pharmacological action to that of metoclopramide, but has a lower side-effect profile. It is available in Europe, and not in the USA.

Cisapride is approved in the USA for the treatment of nocturnal heartburn and is prescribed around the world for heartburn and symptoms of

TABLE 2.4

Medical treatments for GORD

Class and drug	Dose	Endoscopic improvement (%)*
H$_2$-receptor antagonist		
Cimetidine	400 mg, four times a day	~70
Ranitidine	150–300 mg,** twice a day	~80
Famotidine	20–40 mg, twice a day	~80
Nizatidine	150 mg, twice a day	~50
Proton-pump inhibitors		
Omeprazole	20–40 mg, once a day	~90
Lansoprazole	30 mg, once a day	~90
Prokinetic agents		
Metoclopramide	10 mg, four times a day	~70
Cisapride	10 mg, three times a day, or 20 mg, twice a day (UK) 10–20 mg, four times a day (USA)	~70

*Data from Bell and Hunt 1991

**The higher dose may be needed if the patient has erosive changes or is symptomatically resistant to the lower dose

delayed gastric emptying. In the UK, the usual dose is 10 mg, three or four times a day, or 20 mg, twice a day. In the USA, the usual dose is 10–20 mg, four times a day (before meals and at bedtime). It is a peripherally acting 5-HT$_4$ agonist that increases acetylcholine release from the myenteric neurones of the oesophagus and stomach. As a result, it increases the amplitude of oesophageal contractions and LOS pressure. Cisapride also increases the rate of gastric emptying. It is not specific for the oesophagus and the stomach; small bowel and colonic contractions are also stimulated to varying degrees. Side-effects include abdominal cramps, diarrhoea and headache.

Cisapride is associated with an increase in the risk of QT prolongation, torsades de pointes and ventricular dysrhythmia in patients at risk for ventricular dysrhythmia. Also, drugs that increase cisapride blood levels by interfering with cisapride metabolism at the hepatic cytochrome P_{450} 3A4 have a small, but increased, risk of significant cardiac dysrhythmia. As a result, cisapride is contraindicated in combination with erythromycin and other macrolides, antifungal agents, protease inhibitors and the antidepressant drug paroxetine.

Proton-pump inhibitors, such as omeprazole, lansoprazole, pantoprazole and rabeprazole, are the most potent acid-inhibiting agents available. Acid inhibition is significantly greater with this type of drug than with the H_2-receptor antagonists. Recommended doses to achieve greater than 90% healing rates for endoscopically proven oesophagitis are 20 mg, once a day, for omeprazole or 30 mg, once a day, for lansoprazole, or 40 mg, once a day, for pantoprazole or 20 mg, once a day, for rabeprazole, for routine purposes. For resistant cases, 20 mg, twice a day, or 40 mg, once a day, of omeprazole should be given. Proton-pump inhibitors are very effective for healing severe, erosive oesophagitis. Whether they should be first-line treatment for patients with heartburn or used after H_2-receptor antagonists or prokinetic agents have failed to relieve symptoms adequately remains controversial. Long-term use of omeprazole is associated with elevated gastrin levels and chronic atrophic gastritis, but gastric carcinoids or other serious sequelae have not been reported.

Carafate, available in the USA, is a complex carbohydrate in oral suspension that can also be used to provide topical healing for oesophagitis and heartburn.

Stage III. Younger patients requiring high doses of expensive medications to control GORD symptoms may be candidates for surgery. The Nissen fundoplication operation is the most commonly performed surgical procedure for GORD. The gastric fundus is wrapped around itself and the distal oesophagus, and any hiatal hernia is reduced (Figure 2.3). When the operation is successful, over 85% of patients will have no heartburn or regurgitation and medications for GORD symptoms may be reduced or stopped. The procedure decreases the incidence of transient lower oesophageal relaxations and increases LOS pressure. After Nissen fundoplication, a minority of patients may have difficulty with swallowing and/or belching and may suffer 'gas bloat'.

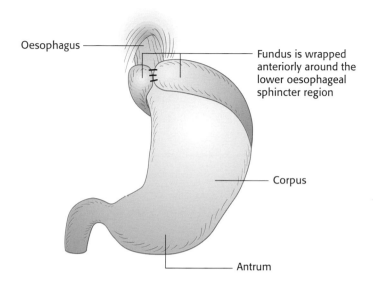

Oesophagus

Fundus is wrapped anteriorly around the lower oesophageal sphincter region

Corpus

Antrum

Figure 2.3 The Nissen fundoplication operation for drug-refractory GORD symptoms.

Nissen fundoplication should not be performed until an oesophageal manometry study has shown low or low-normal LOS pressure. In addition, achalasia, diffuse oesophageal spasm or severe non-specific contractile abnormalities of the oesophageal body should be excluded prior to performing this surgery. Those patients with scleroderma and GORD symptoms should not have a Nissen fundoplication because dysphagia is increased.

If symptoms suggestive of gastroparesis are present, a gastric emptying study should be considered before surgery. The effect of fundoplication on existing gastroparesis has not been studied, but gastroparesis has been reported after fundoplication. Nissen fundoplication can be performed laparoscopically and results appear to be satisfactory and comparable to the open approach when performed by experienced surgeons.

CHAPTER 3
Helicobacter pylori

Although spiral bacteria in the stomach had been reported by numerous observers since the 19th century, it was not until 1982 that Marshall and Warren cultured the organism that was later to be named *Helicobacter pylori* and which today is known to be prevalent worldwide (Figure 3.1). They and others rapidly recognized its close association with gastritis and peptic ulceration; more recently, its aetiological importance in gastric carcinoma and B-cell mucosa-associated lymphoid tissue (MALT) lymphoma has been established (Figure 3.2). There can be few discoveries that have so dramatically changed our understanding and management of such universal diseases.

Bacteriological features

H. pylori is a spiral, flagellate, Gram-negative, micro-aerophilic bacterium. It is uniquely adapted to survive in the hostile environment of the stomach. The bacterium establishes itself by excluding acid from its immediate

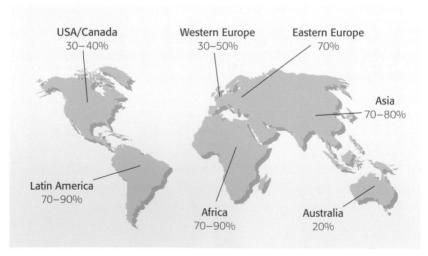

Figure 3.1 *H. pylori* is a ubiquitous organism with highest prevalence rates in the developing world. Reproduced with permission from Marshall BJ. *JAMA* 1995; 274:1064–6. © American Medical Association.

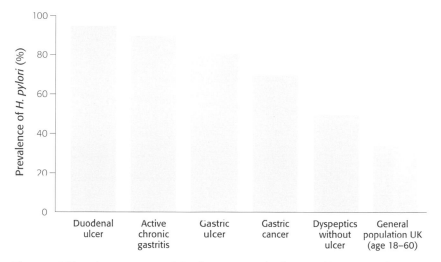

Figure 3.2 There is a strong association between peptic ulcer, gastritis, gastric malignancy and *H. pylori* infection.

surroundings. It does so by converting naturally occurring urea into carbon dioxide and ammonia, and expelling hydrogen ions using its own proton pump.

H. pylori is highly motile, so it is able to exist in both the gastric lumen and mucus gel layer. It also possesses powerful adhesins, by which it attaches firmly to gastric epithelial cells where release of toxins initiates tissue damage and inflammation. It shows considerable diversity of toxin production, which probably explains why certain strains are more strongly associated with gastroduodenal diseases than others.

Infection: when, who and how

Age of infection. In the western world, the prevalence of infection increases with age (Figure 3.3). However, it now seems that rather than being due to a steady acquisition of infection during adult life, this reflects a cohort effect. The elevated level of infection in those who are now elderly is the result of a high incidence of infection when they were young. Similarly, the lower prevalence in today's younger adults is the result of a falling incidence of infection during their childhood and adolescence, probably as a result of improved socioeconomic conditions. In contrast, the overwhelming majority of the population of developing countries continues to become infected

27

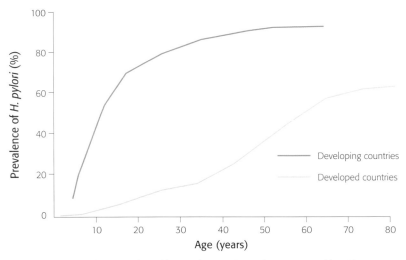

Figure 3.3 In the developed world, prevalence of *H. pylori* rises steadily with age, whereas the great majority of the population in developing countries is infected before the age of 20. Reproduced with permission from Northfield *et al. Helicobacter pylori* infection. © 1993 Kluwer.

before they are 20 years old (Figure 3.3). Regardless of geography, risk of acquisition is greatest during childhood, though up to 0.5% of adults in industrialized countries still become infected annually.

Socioeconomic factors. In developed and developing countries, the prevalence of *H. pylori* infection is directly proportional to the level of socioeconomic deprivation, whether measured by education, income, occupation or living conditions. Children are most vulnerable and act as vectors of infection between adults.

Source and route of infection. It has been suggested that domestic and abattoir-slaughtered animals might act as a possible reservoir for human infection. As for other gastrointestinal infections, drinking water in the developing world is also a potential source of infection. Direct, person-to-person spread is suggested by the increased prevalence of infection in residential institutions.

Isolation of *H. pylori* from dental plaque and vomit supports the contention that oral–oral transmission is important. However, the organism retains viability in faeces and the faecal–oral route of infection is potentially more universal. Sources and routes of *H. pylori* infection are shown in Table 3.1.

Diseases associated with infection

Acute gastritis. Initial infection of the stomach may be asymptomatic, but some patients experience an illness lasting 1–2 weeks that includes epigastric pain, vomiting, nausea and occasionally pyrexia. This phase is accompanied by achlorhydria, which may take several months to resolve. Some patients spontaneously clear the organism, but the majority remain chronically infected.

Chronic gastritis. The severity and distribution of chronic *H. pylori* infection is likely to depend upon bacterial characteristics, host response and environmental factors (Table 3.2). Interaction between these factors results in three distinct patterns of gastritis and subsequent morbidity (Figure 3.4).

Pan gastritis patients have normal parietal cell mass but a pre-morbid reduced response to gastrin (Figure 3.4a). *H. pylori* is able to infect the body of the stomach as well as the antrum because, unlike in duodenal ulcer patients, there is no excess acid secretion from this part of the stomach. Despite elevated levels of serum gastrin following infection, excess acid

TABLE 3.1

Possible sources and routes of transmission of *H. pylori*

Hosts

- Primary
  - humans

- Reservoir
  - cats (proven)
  - pigs (suspected)
  - monkey (proven)

Routes and modes of contamination

- Faecal–oral?
  - uncooked vegetables
  - surface (or well) water swimming/ingestion

- Oral–oral
  - vomitus
  - kissing

TABLE 3.2

Factors that may influence the consequences of *H. pylori* infection

Bacterial characteristics

- Initial bacterial load
- Toxin production (*cagA* and *vacA* are associated with ulcer and gastric cancer)
- Adhesins

Host response

- HLA type and expression on gastric epithelium
- IgA response relative to IgM and IgG response
- Variable release of prostaglandins and leukotrienes
- Parietal cell mass and acid secretion
- Duodenogastric reflux
- Vascularity of gastric mucosa

Environmental factors

- Age at time of infection
- Dietary factors (excess salt and nitrates, vitamin C and E deficiencies)
- Non-steroidal anti-inflammatory drugs

HLA, human leukocyte antigen

secretion does not occur because parietal cell function is impaired further by *H. pylori* infection of the gastric body. The great majority of these patients remain asymptomatic.

Antral gastritis. This is associated with duodenal ulcer (Figure 3.4b). *H. pylori* infection is restricted to the antrum in those patients with a pre-morbid, genetically determined, increased parietal cell mass in the corpus (where colonization is prevented by elevated acid secretion). Infection of the antrum leads to hypergastrinaemia (see Duodenal ulcer, page 42), which stimulates the increased parietal cell mass to secrete excess acid that, in turn, induces gastric metaplasia in the duodenal mucosa allowing *H. pylori* colonization.

Gastritis of the corpus. This is associated with gastric ulcer and adenocarcinoma (Figure 3.4c). Exposure to *H. pylori* in early childhood

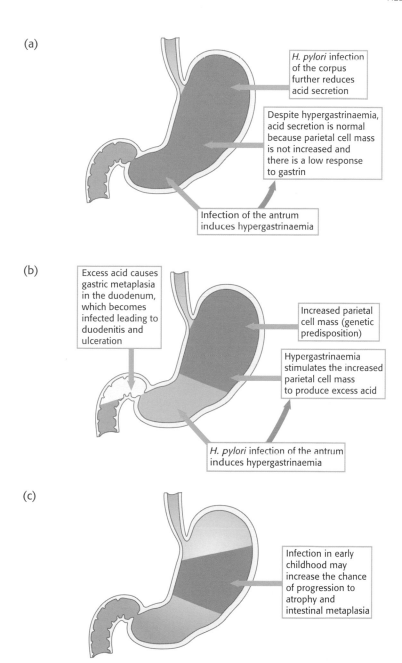

Figure 3.4 The three distinct patterns of gastritis: (a) pan gastritis; (b) antral gastritis; and (c) gastritis of the corpus.

31

may predispose patients to infection of the gastric body with sparing of the antrum, resulting in atrophy of the parietal cell area, reduced acid secretion and secondary hypergastrinaemia. Atrophy and achlorhydria can potentially enhance ulcerogenic co-factors such as non-steroidal anti-inflammatory drugs (NSAIDs) and refluxed bile. Intestinal metaplasia accompanies severe and long standing gastric atrophy, which are known predisposing factors for carcinoma of the stomach. Achlorhydria encourages bacterial overgrowth, which enhances production of carcinogens.

Duodenal and gastric ulcer. The role of *H. pylori* in the pathogenesis of duodenal and gastric ulcer is described in Chapter 4.

Gastric cancer. Worldwide, gastric carcinoma is the second most common cancer, affecting up to 10 million people annually. *H. pylori* was designated a class one carcinogen by the World Health Organization in 1994. Epidemiological evidence and the fact that *H. pylori* is accompanied by mucosal changes conducive to carcinogenesis support the association of *H. pylori* infection with gastric cancer (Table 3.3).

Potential for prevention. It seems likely that prevention or treatment of infection during childhood is likely to have the greatest impact on reducing the subsequent development of gastric cancer. The effect of improved living

TABLE 3.3

Evidence to support an association between gastric cancer and *H. pylori*

- There is worldwide correlation between prevalence of *H. pylori* and incidence of gastric cancer
- Gastric cancer has declined in parallel with the rate of *H. pylori* infection
- Infected individuals have an increased risk of gastric cancer
- *H. pylori* causes gastric atrophy and intestinal metaplasia that precede dysplasia and neoplasia
- Corporal gastritis increases gastric pH and reduces secretion of vitamin C, predisposing to bacterial proliferation and production of carcinogenic nitrosocompounds

standards is already evident in industrialized countries. Childhood screening combined with eradication therapy may further reduce the risk, though this strategy has less potential in the developing world where re-infection rates are high. Whether eradication therapy in adults prevents progression of carcinogenesis remains to be proved. In worldwide terms, a significant impact on gastric cancer is only likely to occur with improved living standards and possibly vaccination.

Gastric lymphoma. In some individuals, *H. pylori* infection induces a proliferation of gastric mucosal lymphocytes. In a very small minority, this progresses to true lymphoma – so-called MALT lymphoma. In most people, the lesion regresses following *H. pylori* eradication.

Functional dyspepsia. The role of *H. pylori* in dyspepsia in the absence of ulcer disease is uncertain. Based on the available evidence, summarized below, it is probably only of primary importance in a minority of patients suffering from this heterogeneous disorder.

- Only a minority of those infected have symptoms.
- *H. pylori*-positive patients have symptoms comparable to those of *H. pylori*-negative patients.
- Although dyspeptic patients have a higher prevalence of infection than non-dyspeptics, the control individuals used in many studies have been inappropriate.
- Some patients improve after eradication therapy, but results are generally disappointing compared with those achieved in patients with ulcer disease.

Nevertheless, future research may identify certain subgroups of *H. pylori*-infected, functional dyspeptics that might benefit from eradication therapy.

Methods of detection

The advantages, disadvantages and application of these tests in clinical practice are summarized in Table 3.4.

Rapid urease test. This is usually the *Campylobacter*-like organism (CLO) test, which is performed during endoscopy. Infected biopsies result in

33

TABLE 3.4

Tests used in the detection of *H. pylori*

Test	Sensitivity (%)	Specificity (%)	Advantages
Rapid urease test	≤ 95	95	Rapid result
Histology	85	100	Very specific
Culture	95	100	Establishes antibiotic sensitivity
Urea breath test	97	95	Non-invasive
Serology	70–90	50–90	Inexpensive

ammonia generation and raised pH, changing the indicator from yellow to pink. It is a reliable, routine method of establishing *H. pylori* status.

Histology and culture tend to be reserved for clinical trials. However, culture is also used in areas where antibiotic resistance is common, as antibiotic sensitivities can be determined at the same time.

Urea breath test (UBT) is a non-invasive test for establishing current *H. pylori* status (Figure 3.5) and is particularly useful when there is doubt following eradication therapy. The validity of the test is significantly impaired if it is used less than 28 days after completing *H. pylori* eradication or within 14 days of stopping a proton-pump inhibitor.

Serological tests are valuable for population screening, but have little use in post-eradication evaluation because antibody titres may take several months to fall. Laboratory-based tests have better specificity and sensitivity compared with tests promoted for office use.

Who should be treated?

The Maastricht consensus meeting, in 1996, recommended *H. pylori* eradication:

* for patients with gastric and duodenal ulcers, including those with a past history of confirmed disease

Disadvantages	Application
Requires endoscopy	Routine during endoscopy
Requires endoscopy and is expensive	Supplements rapid urease test
Expensive and delay in obtaining results	In areas of high antibiotic resistance
Expensive	To check eradication
Poor specificity (laboratory tests are superior to 'office' kits)	Screening

- for patients with severe gastritis (erosive or atrophic disease)
- for patients with MALT lymphoma
- following resection for early gastric cancer.

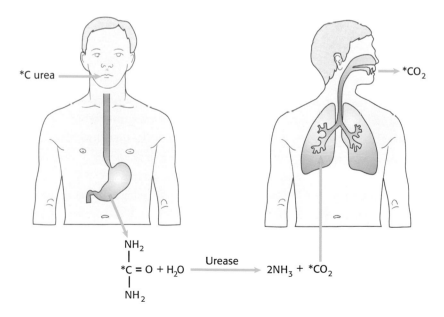

Figure 3.5 The urea breath test. Urea containing a carbon isotope label is given to the patient. If *H. pylori* is present in the stomach, the urea is metabolized and labelled carbon dioxide is detectable in the patient's breath.

The meeting also proposed that eradication therapy should be considered in other situations even though irrefutable evidence to support its use is unavailable. These include:

- functional dyspepsia – presumably because symptomatic relief occurs in a minority of *H. pylori*-positive patients without overt mucosal disease
- non-steroidal anti-inflammatory drug use – it is impossible to know which of the two aetiological factors is primarily to blame for an ulcer found in an *H. pylori*-positive patient taking an NSAID
- family history of gastric cancer – possible predisposing genetic factors may increase the risk of *H. pylori*-induced carcinogenesis
- long-term proton-pump inhibitor therapy – *H. pylori* has a tendency to migrate from the antrum to the gastric corpus during long-term therapy with these agents, leading to atrophic gastritis and the subsequent potential risk of gastric ulcer or cancer. Atrophy in the corpus could be prevented by prior eradication, but such a policy has yet to be adopted widely.

Currently, eradication therapy is not recommended for:

- patients with GORD
- asymptomatic subjects.

Patients with GORD. Eradication of *H. pylori* has the potential to exacerbate symptoms in some patients with GORD and coexisting gastritis of the corpus because gastric acid secretion increases after inflammation in the parietal cell area heals. In others, control of symptoms with a proton-pump inhibitor may become less effective because these drugs appear to have greater efficacy in the presence of gastritis than when the stomach is healthy.

Asymptomatic patients. Treating asymptomatic patients may potentially prevent progression to peptic ulcer and possibly even reverse pre-malignant gastric mucosal disease. However, some previously asymptomatic patients will develop antibiotic-induced gastrointestinal problems. There is also a risk that indiscriminate use of antibiotics might encourage resistant strains. Furthermore, it has been argued that some strains of *H. pylori* may actually confer a health benefit.

Once aware that they are infected, many people, even in the absence of symptoms, will 'demand' eradication therapy and such demands are often difficult to resist.

Eradication regimens

H. pylori eradication rates of over 90% are now readily achievable. The most extensively studied and consistently effective regimens consist of a proton-pump inhibitor and two antibiotics given for 7 days. Comparable results have also been reported with ranitidine bismuth citrate in combination with clarithromycin and metronidazole or amoxycillin (Table 3.5).

In areas where metronidazole resistance is common, it is logical to use a regimen without this antibiotic or to ascertain bacterial sensitivities before prescribing.

With gastric ulcer, successful eradication can be confirmed at repeat endoscopy. For the majority of other patients, eradication may be assumed if symptoms resolve. For those who continue to be symptomatic and for

TABLE 3.5

Recommended 7-day, triple-therapy regimens

A

Omeprazole, 20 mg, twice a day **or** lansoprazole, 30 mg, twice a day **or** pantoprazole, 40 mg, twice a day **or** ranitidine bismuth citrate, 400 mg, twice a day
PLUS
Metronidazole, 400 mg, twice a day
PLUS
Clarithromycin, 250 mg, twice a day

B

Omeprazole, 20 mg, twice a day **or** lansoprazole, 30 mg, twice a day **or** pantoprazole, 40 mg, twice a day **or** ranitidine bismuth citrate, 400 mg, twice a day
PLUS
Amoxycillin, 1 g, twice a day
PLUS
Clarithromycin, 500 mg, twice a day

C

Omeprazole, 40 mg, once a day **or** lansoprazole, 30 mg, twice a day
PLUS
Amoxycillin, 500 mg, three times a day
PLUS
Metronidazole, 400 mg, three times a day

TABLE 3.6

At-risk patients in whom eradication should be confirmed

- History of complicated ulcer
- Long-term anticoagulant medication
- Frail patients with serious concomitant disease

patients for whom persistent infection would be potentially hazardous (Table 3.6), the UBT is an appropriate means of confirming eradication. When infection persists despite satisfactory compliance, a further course of triple therapy extended for 10 or 14 days should be tried. When proton-pump inhibitor-based triple therapy has failed, an alternative approach would be to use a bismuth-containing regimen (Table 3.7).

So-called 'dual therapy' using a proton-pump inhibitor and a single antibiotic achieves unsatisfactory eradication rates and may encourage bacterial resistance. It is **not** recommended.

TABLE 3.7

Recommended 14-day regimen after proton-pump inhibitor-based triple-therapy failure

A proton-pump inhibitor, twice a day, with tri-potassium di-citrato bismuthate, 120 mg, twice a day **or** ranitidine bismuth citrate, 400 mg, twice a day
PLUS
Metronidazole, 400 mg, three times a day
PLUS
Tetracycline, 500 mg, three times a day

CHAPTER 4

Peptic ulcer

The exact incidence and prevalence of peptic ulcer have always been uncertain because of the remitting and relapsing nature of the disease and the erratic investigation of dyspepsia. A decade ago, the lifetime risk of peptic ulcer in the UK was approximately 10%, and about 500 000 new cases were diagnosed in the USA each year.

Duodenal ulcer is three to four times more common than gastric ulcer. In the past, the disease predominated in men but the male:female ratio now approximates to unity, particularly in the elderly (Figure 4.1).

Although overall admission rates have fallen in both the USA and the UK, the number of hospitalizations for ulcer complications has risen. Every year, approximately 4500 people in the UK die from peptic ulcer; of these, more than 90% are over the age of 60 years (Figure 4.2). Without control of the disease, 15% of ulcer patients may experience haemorrhage within 10 years of diagnosis and it has been estimated that 15% of those who bleed eventually die as a result of their ulcer. Until it was recently established that we could change their natural history by *H. pylori* eradication, duodenal and gastric ulcers were chronic diseases with annual relapse rates of around 80% and 40%, respectively.

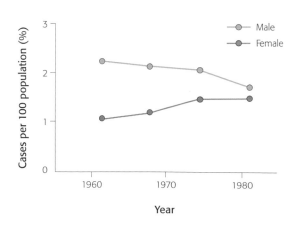

Figure 4.1

The prevalence of peptic ulcer has decreased in males and increased in females. Data from Kurata JH. *Gastroenterology* 1989;96:569–80 and Kurata JH *et al*. *Am J Public Health* 1985;75:625–9.

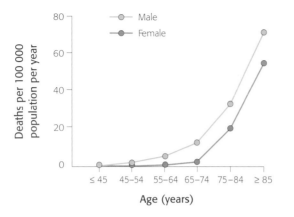

Figure 4.2

Mortality in peptic ulcer disease increases with age. Many older patients with ulcer disease have concomitant cardiorespiratory disease.

In the western world, the incidence of peptic ulcer has been in decline for the past 30 years as a result of the falling prevalence of *H. pylori* infection. It seems likely that this decline will be accelerated further by the widespread adoption of bacterial eradication, though the increasing use of NSAIDs may be counteractive. By far the most common sites of peptic ulcer are the first part of the duodenum and the stomach (Figure 4.3). Ulcers may also occur in the oesophagus as a consequence of gastro-oesophageal reflux (Chapter 2) and, very rarely, at gastroenteric stoma following gastric surgery or in association with a Meckel's diverticulum.

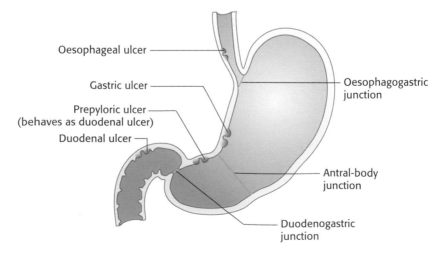

Figure 4.3 Peptic ulcers commonly occur adjacent to mucosal junctions.

Pathogenesis

H. pylori. The traditional view is that peptic ulceration occurs when gastro-duodenal mucosa breaks down under the erosive effect of gastric acid and pepsin. Although aetiopathogenic processes between gastric and duodenal ulcers differ significantly, it is now accepted that *H. pylori* infection is a common causative factor (Table 4.1). The mechanisms by which *H. pylori* causes peptic ulceration depend on the disturbance of acid secretion and the direct effect of bacterial inflammation on the gastroduodenal mucosa.

TABLE 4.1

Aetiological risk factors and special features of peptic ulcer

H. pylori

- Infection is found in 95% of duodenal ulcer and 80% of gastric ulcer patients

NSAIDs

- Counteract the protective effects of prostaglandins
- Approximately 20% of regular users have ulceration of the gastroduodenal mucosa
- Risk of ulceration is increased by concomitant steroid therapy, smoking and possibly *H. pylori* infection
- Typical pain is often absent
- Presentation with anaemia and acute haemorrhage is common
- Toxicity varies according to drug: azapropazone and piroxicam appear to be particularly toxic, ibuprofen less so

Smoking

- Smokers have an increased prevalence of ulcers, delayed healing and increased incidence of complications

Steroids

- Long-term use of corticosteroids may increase risk of peptic ulcer, but the risk is lower than that associated with NSAID therapy

Genetic

- Siblings are 2.5 times more likely to have an ulcer compared with controls
- Genetic studies may have been confounded by familial transmission of *H. pylori*

Duodenal ulcer. In patients who progress to duodenal ulceration, *H. pylori* infection is confined mainly to the gastric antrum. The mucosa in this portion of the stomach contains gastrin-producing G cells and somatostatin-secreting D cells. Gastrin secretion in response to food stimulates parietal cells in the body of the stomach to produce acid. Somatostatin is secreted in the presence of excess acid. It inhibits gastrin release, thus preventing excessive acid secretion.

H. pylori infection of the antrum leads to the suppression of somatostatin release from D cells. This causes a rise in gastrin and, in turn, increased secretion of acid by parietal cells, the numbers of which are increased in duodenal ulcer patients (Figure 4.4). This excess acid passes into the duodenum, where it induces gastric metaplasia in the duodenal mucosa. *H. pylori*, which is incapable of infecting healthy duodenal mucosa, now colonizes the patches of gastric metaplasia, which leads to duodenitis and ulceration.

Gastric ulcer. The predominant site of *H. pylori* infection is the body of the stomach, where it leads to atrophy of the mucosa and reduction of acid

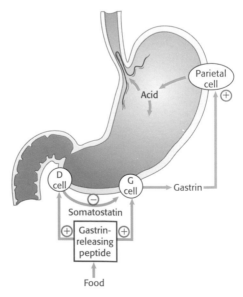

Figure 4.4 The control of acid secretion and the relationship between G, D and parietal cells.

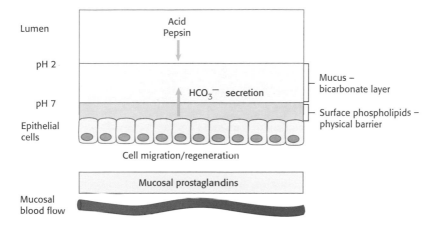

Figure 4.5 Maintenance of mucosal defence. The mucus layer retains bicarbonate, which is secreted by epithelial cells and neutralizes acid as it penetrates from the lumen. The epithelial cells form a second line of defence. Prostaglandin secretion suppresses acid secretion and increases mucosal blood flow, which is essential for epithelial integrity.

secretion. These conditions predispose to ulceration in the stomach, but other factors that have yet to be fully identified or confirmed must also be involved.

Mucosal defence

The maintenance of mucosal defence (Figure 4.5) depends on many factors, including:

- the structure of the epithelial surface and its ability to regenerate and repair
- secretion of water, mucus and bicarbonate
- mucosal blood flow.

At the mucosal level, the pathogenic processes that result in ulceration have still to be clarified. Mucosal integrity is, however, compromised by factors such as *H. pylori* toxins, NSAIDs, corticosteroids and smoking (see Table 4.1).

Gastroduodenal dysmotility

Excessive acidification of the duodenal bulb and the mucosal damage that results due to uncoordinated and rapid gastric emptying occur in some patients with duodenal ulcer. These factors may be the predominant pathogenic mechanism in non-*H. pylori*/non-NSAID duodenal ulcers.

Duodenogastric reflux of bile and pancreatic enzymes may be supplementary aetiological factors in gastric ulcer.

Zollinger-Ellison syndrome

Zollinger-Ellison (ZE) syndrome is a rare cause of duodenal ulcer. It is characterized by a very high basal rate of gastric acid secretion due, in the majority of patients, to a gastrin-producing tumour of the pancreas. In others, the tumour is found in other abdominal organs. Rarely, the syndrome results from hyperplasia of G cells in the antrum. The features of ZE syndrome are summarized in Table 4.2.

Diagnosis

Pain localized to the epigastrium is the characteristic feature of peptic ulcer. More rarely, pain occurs in the hypochondria or around the umbilicus. Radiation retrosternally or to the back is often experienced. It is usually described as 'gnawing' or 'knife-like'. Sometimes patients describe a feeling of severe hunger. The pain can last from several minutes to a few hours. Increasing intensity of pain does not indicate incipient perforation or haemorrhage, but may be the result of penetration into the pancreas. Without treatment, pain tends to occur in bouts, which persist for a few weeks, followed by remissions, which may last for several months. Pain in the early hours is a feature of duodenal ulcer; it is unrelated to eating in at least 50% of patients. Consistent relief with antacids is frequently reported.

TABLE 4.2

Features of Zollinger-Ellison syndrome

- Absence of *H. pylori* infection
- Failure of ulcer to heal with routine acid suppression
- Ulceration beyond the first part of the duodenum
- Accompanying diarrhoea or steatorrhoea
- Response to tumour resection or high-dose proton-pump inhibitor therapy

Vomiting and reflux. Although uncommon, vomiting that relieves pain is a sensitive indicator of duodenal ulcer. Heartburn and regurgitation also occur frequently.

Examination

The only physical sign of uncomplicated peptic ulcer is epigastric tenderness. The presence of this sign does not discriminate an ulcer from other abdominal diseases.

Importantly, it is not possible to distinguish between gastric and duodenal ulcers on the basis of clinical features alone.

Investigations

Upper gastrointestinal endoscopy is the first choice for patients with symptoms suggestive of peptic ulcer. It is more accurate than a barium meal, allows histological diagnosis and establishes *H. pylori* status. A barium meal should be reserved for patients stating a preference for this procedure or when endoscopy is technically impossible. However, if an initial barium meal shows gastric ulcer, it should be followed by UGI endoscopy to exclude malignancy.

Biochemical tests. Anaemia due to occult bleeding should always be excluded in ulcer disease. In ZE syndrome, the serum gastrin level will be greatly elevated and the basal level of acid secretion will be high. Elevated serum gastrin levels are also found in patients taking acid-suppressant drugs and those with pernicious anaemia.

Management

H. pylori-**associated ulcers.** Bacterial eradication therapy is the first choice for newly diagnosed duodenal and gastric ulcers following confirmation of *H. pylori* infection (Chapter 3). It is undoubtedly the most cost-effective means of ulcer management, because successful eradication dramatically reduces recurrence (Figure 4.6).

It is also acceptable to offer eradication therapy to patients with a past history of confirmed chronic ulcer disease, even when *H. pylori* status has not been established. Some physicians, nevertheless, prefer to confirm infection by serology or UBT.

(a)

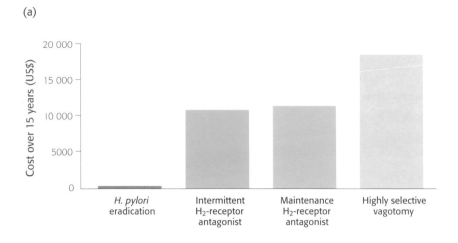

(b)

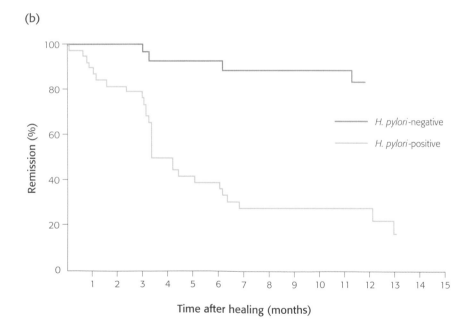

Figure 4.6 (a) Predicted costs of duodenal ulcer management strategies over 15 years (data from Sonnenberg A and Townsend WF 1995); (b) eradication of *H. pylori* dramatically reduces the recurrence of duodenal ulcer. Reproduced with permission from Calam J. *Clinician's Guide to Helicobacter Pylori*, 1996.

Ulcers heal following successful eradication; prolonged courses of either H_2-receptor antagonists or proton-pump inhibitors are not usually required for uncomplicated disease. However, some patients continue to use them for a few weeks if symptoms persist temporarily.

Confirmation of healing. Repeat endoscopy is unnecessary for patients with uncomplicated duodenal ulcer. Resolution of symptoms can be taken as confirmation of eradication and healing. In contrast, gastric ulcer healing must be confirmed by repeat endoscopy, which in addition provides the means of reassessing *H. pylori* status.

For duodenal ulcer presenting with haemorrhage or perforation, current practice is to suppress acid secretion for 4 weeks, in addition to giving eradication therapy, to enhance healing. Furthermore, many gastroenterologists recommend endoscopic confirmation of healing and bacterial clearance for this patient group. Successful eradication virtually eliminates the risk of recurrent bleeding.

Persistent symptoms. Dyspepsia that persists after eradication therapy for ulcer disease is rarely due to failed bacterial clearance or continuing ulceration, as eradication rates of over 90% are now readily achievable. Residual symptoms are usually due to coexisting disorders, such as reflux disease or functional dyspepsia.

In this circumstance, the UBT is the most sensitive and convenient means of excluding persistent infection. If failed eradication is confirmed, a further antibacterial course should be given (Chapter 2). Failure to eradicate *H. pylori* in ulcer disease leaves the patient at risk of recurrence and potential complications. In this situation, long-term maintenance with acid suppression is the logical means of disease control.

NSAID-associated ulcers. When the NSAID is withdrawn, ulcers heal rapidly on standard acid-suppressant therapy. If the NSAID has to be continued, ulcer healing is slowed when H_2-receptor antagonists are used at routine dosage. Proton-pump inhibition is therefore preferable. Concomitant prophylactic protective therapy should be considered in certain NSAID users (Table 4.3); proton-pump inhibitors are more effective than H_2-receptor antagonists or misoprostol.

TABLE 4.3

Patients using NSAIDs for whom prophylactic proton-pump inhibitor therapy should be considered

- Patients with previous history of significant dyspepsia
- Patients with previous history of ulcer, particularly with complications
- Smokers
- Patients receiving a high-dose NSAID or concomitant steroid therapy
- Patients given NSAIDs known to be associated with a higher incidence of gastrointestinal complications, such as piroxicam or azapropazone

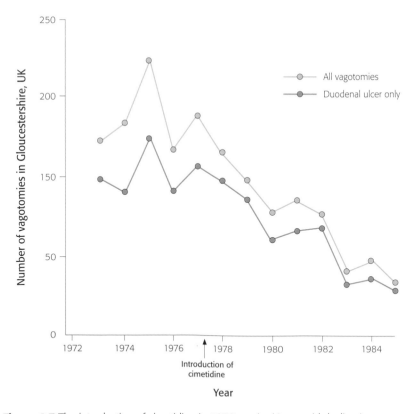

Figure 4.7 The introduction of cimetidine in 1976 resulted in a rapid decline in operations for duodenal ulcer in Gloucestershire, UK. Reproduced from Gear MWL, 1986.

There is some evidence that *H. pylori* infection may increase the incidence of dyspepsia and ulceration in NSAID users. However, it is not current practice to establish *H. pylori* status or to offer eradication prior to NSAID therapy because there is, at present, no established proof that this would significantly reduce the incidence of NSAID-induced disease.

Non-*H. pylori*, non-NSAID ulcers. A small minority of chronic peptic ulcers are not associated with either *H. pylori* or NSAID use. They are suitably controlled by prolonged acid-suppressant therapy.

Endoscopic management of acute haemorrhage. Acute haemorrhage from an ulcer accounts for 2500 deaths annually in the UK. In the USA, the reported mortality rate from acute UGI haemorrhage is 5–14%, and depends on variables such as age and comorbid conditions.

Early endoscopic examination allows investigation of the bleeding site, which can then be treated by laser, heater probe or injection of adrenaline and sclerosant. Such intervention reduces rates of re-bleeding, transfusion requirements, surgical referral and hospitalization time.

Surgery. Increasing use of pharmacological control of gastric acid secretion has accelerated the decline of surgical management of uncomplicated peptic ulcer (Figure 4.7) and it has become virtually obsolete since the introduction of *H. pylori* eradication. The most common indication for surgical intervention is gastric ulcer that fails to heal on medical treatment. This raises the suspicion of undiagnosed malignancy, which is found in approximately 2% of gastric ulcers originally considered to be benign. Most surgeons now opt for minimal intervention when operating for bleeding or perforation because the disease can be managed subsequently by *H. pylori* eradication or long-term acid suppression.

CHAPTER 5
Carcinoma of the oesophagus and stomach

Although UGI symptoms suggestive of oesophageal or gastric cancer naturally raise concern in general practice, malignancy is in fact a relatively rare cause of dyspepsia in most of the developed world. Approximately only 3% of all patients investigated by UGI endoscopy in the UK have carcinoma of the oesophagus or stomach.

The incidence of malignant disease increases with age. A survey, performed by Michael Lancaster Smith, of 9000 unselected consecutive endoscopies, revealed that:

- the incidences of oesophageal and gastric carcinomas were 1 per 1000 and 1 per 650, respectively, in patients under 45 years of age
- only 1.2% of all patients with carcinoma of the oesophagus and 1.7% of those with stomach cancer were below the age of 45.

Carcinoma of the oesophagus

The incidence of oesophageal cancer varies widely; for example, in some areas of China and Iran, it exceeds that of western Europe and North America by a factor of 10. In the USA, incidence is three to four times greater in blacks than whites. The annual incidence in the UK is approximately 8 per 100 000. The increasing incidence of distal carcinoma in the developed world during the past 30 years is thought to be related to severe gastro-oesophageal reflux.

Aetiopathogenesis. The aetiological factors involved include:
- smoking
- heavy consumption of alcohol
- diet (fungal contamination of food, vitamin, iron and zinc deficiencies, high nitrite and nitrate intake)
- Barrett's oesophagus/severe gastro-oesophageal reflux
- achalasia
- coeliac disease
- tylosis (familial hyperkeratosis).

Approximately 70% of oesophageal cancers are squamous cell lesions and 30% adenocarcinomas; the latter predominate distally. Oesophageal cancer invades the mediastinum and may also extend into the proximal stomach. Lymphatic spread may involve the supraclavicular and intra-abdominal nodes.

Diagnosis and management. The predominant symptom is progressive dysphagia, usually accompanied by some degree of anorexia and weight loss. Upper gastrointestinal endoscopy is the most accurate means of confirming the diagnosis. Staging of the disease by CT, MRI or endoscopic ultrasound enables selection of potentially curable patients for radical surgery. The overall 5-year survival in such cases is 10–20%.

Radiotherapy is preferred for upper-third lesions and may be curative. Elsewhere radiotherapy is usually palliative. The primary objective of palliation is to maintain swallowing. New chemotherapeutic regimens have also shown encouraging results in terms of palliation. Other palliative measures include:

- regular endoscopic dilatation
- endoscopically or radiologically positioned stents
- tumour ablation with alcohol or laser.

Improved outcome in the future will depend upon earlier investigation and screening of high-risk patients, such as those with dysplastic Barrett's mucosa and possibly those with severe gastro-oesophageal reflux.

Carcinoma of the stomach

Prevalence rates for carcinoma of the stomach vary widely throughout the world. It is particularly common in Japan, Chile, Finland and parts of China. In the developed world, the incidence of cancers in the distal stomach has fallen dramatically during the past 50 years. In contrast, there has been a steady increase in the frequency of proximal carcinomas (Figure 5.1). In the UK, a family physician with an average list will see one new case every 2 years.

Aetiopathogenesis. The aetiology of the disease involves both genetic and environmental factors (Table 5.1), but there is now little doubt that *H. pylori* is the most important contributor (see Chapter 3). The reduced

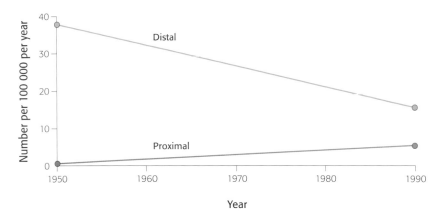

Figure 5.1 Incidence of distal and proximal gastric cancer in The Netherlands. Reproduced with permission from Kuipers EJ. *Aliment Pharmacol Ther* 1999;13 (Suppl 1):3–11.

incidence of distal stomach cancer in developed countries has been attributed to the ever-decreasing prevalence of *H. pylori* gastritis. Carcinomas occur in any area of the stomach and may be ulcerative, polypoid and occasionally diffusely infiltrative (linitis plastica). The regional lymph nodes and peritoneum are sites of local spread, with secondary deposits common in the liver and more distant metastases occurring in bone and lung.

Diagnosis and management. The clinical features of gastric cancer include:
- epigastric pain
- anorexia
- weight loss
- vomiting
- dysphagia
- anaemia.

Ascites, hepatomegaly and supraclavicular lymphadenopathy are signs of advanced disease. Diagnosis is confirmed by endoscopy and pre-operative staging by CT and laparoscopy.

In Japan, where the incidence of stomach cancer is high, screening programmes detect disease at an early stage and 5-year survival rates have risen to 40%. Unfortunately, in the UK, despite the widespread availability

TABLE 5.1

Aetiological factors for carcinoma of the stomach

- *H. pylori* gastritis
- Autoimmune atrophic gastritis – pernicious anaemia
- Dietary factors (pickled food, low vitamin/high salt intake, smoked food)
- High nitrate ingestion (contaminated water)
- Previous partial gastrectomy
- Blood group A

of open-access endoscopy, only 50% of patients have resectable tumours and 5-year survival rates range from 7 to 16%.

Adjuvant chemotherapeutic regimens are under investigation and appear to extend survival.

CHAPTER 6

Functional dyspepsia

Functional dyspepsia refers to discomfort or pain centred in the epigastrium; it may be 'ulcer-like' or 'dysmotility-like'. Ulcer-like dyspepsia is a burning epigastric discomfort or pain that often occurs at night and improves after eating. Dysmotility-like dyspepsia encompasses a sensation of fullness, nausea or bloating, and vomiting. Symptoms are typically worse in the postprandial period, and the condition described is often referred to as 'dysmotility-like dyspepsia'.

The word 'functional' indicates that common or uncommon structural, biochemical or infectious agents have been excluded as a cause of the dyspepsia symptoms. As described in Chapter 1, uninvestigated symptoms may be due to many causes. In the absence of alarm symptoms, empirical treatment often resolves the symptoms and they do not return.

However, if alarm symptoms are present or if empirical treatment of a reasonable duration does not relieve the symptoms, the patient should undergo investigation. A more specific diagnosis benefits both patient and physician, leading to:

- a better understanding of the patient's symptoms
- an appreciation of the prognosis for the symptoms
- more specific and rational therapies.

Here, an approach to the diagnosis and treatment of functional dyspepsia that begins when the common diagnoses responsible for dyspepsia symptoms have been excluded and the symptoms remain unexplained is reviewed.

Epidemiology

Dyspepsia symptoms are very common and affect 7–40% of various populations. Many patients with mild symptoms do not seek medical attention. The precise number of patients seeking medical care is unknown due to variables in classification. It is clear, however, that in many patients who undergo investigation for dyspepsia symptoms, no specific abnormalities are found. For example, approximately 30% of patients undergoing UGI endoscopy for dyspepsia symptoms have normal endoscopic evaluations. Therefore, from a gastroenterologist's viewpoint, approximately 30% of patients with these non-specific dyspepsia symptoms have functional dyspepsia, provided other causes, such as biliary and pancreatic disease or irritable bowel syndrome, have been excluded.

The definition of functional dyspepsia has been troublesome for many years – dyspepsia literally means 'bad digestion'. The problem stems from the fact that the term is poorly understood by physicians and patients alike – patients do not complain of 'dyspepsia'. Furthermore, the patient may have a difficult time describing the uncomfortable abdominal sensations that they experience after a meal. When physicians try to communicate about dyspepsia, the term is often confused with GORD, heartburn, peptic ulcers, and conditions of mucosal inflammation or ulceration of the oesophagus, stomach and/or duodenum.

When standard tests, such as radiographic studies of the UGI tract and upper endoscopy, exclude the common causes of dyspepsia symptoms, disorders of gastric neuromusculature (motility) should be diagnosed and treated appropriately (see below). Gastric neuromuscular abnormalities are abnormalities of motility or the neuromuscular functions of the stomach and duodenum. They include disorders of:

- fundic and antral contractility and relaxation
- gastric myoelectrical activity
- gastric emptying
- visceral hypersensitivities related to the stomach.

Pathophysiology

Normal postprandial gastroduodenal motility. Myenteric neurones of the enteric nervous system are organized in plexi between the muscle layers. The fundus relaxes after each swallow via non-adrenergic, non-cholinergic neural pathways that probably involve nitric oxide. The fundus and proximal body of the stomach relax to receive ingested food, a process called receptive relaxation (Figure 6.1), allowing the stomach to accommodate the volume of ingested food without producing excessive intragastric pressure.

In humans, the gastric peristaltic waves that move food to the gastric body and antrum occur at a rate of 3 per minute (Figure 6.1). Food is mixed with acid and pepsin until the particles (now under 1 mm in size) are in a nutrient suspension called chyme. Waves of antral peristaltic contraction

55

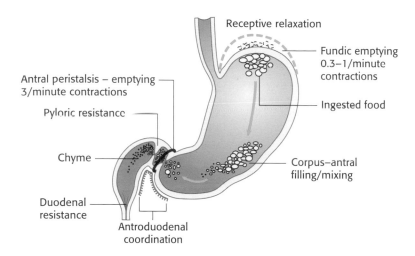

Figure 6.1 Gastric neuromuscular activity in response to a solid meal.

empty 3–4 ml of chyme into the duodenum. Gastric emptying requires coordination between the antrum, pylorus and duodenal motility.

Normal gastric emptying of solids includes a lag phase lasting 30–45 minutes, depending on the calorie content of the meal, and a linear phase of emptying during which the stomach steadily empties the meal over 2–4 hours, depending on the energy density of the food.

Coordination of gastric peristaltic contractions is by gastric slow waves or pacesetter potentials (Figure 6.2). Pacesetter potentials originate on the greater curvature of the stomach near the junction of the fundus and the proximal corpus. They are electrical depolarization and repolarization wave fronts that migrate circumferentially and distally towards the pylorus at a frequency of 3 cycles per minute (range 2.5–3.7 cpm). The 3-cpm pacesetter potential controls the normal gastric peristaltic waves that occur at 3 contractions per minute.

Gastric pacesetter potentials do not produce strong gastric contractions. Circular muscle contraction occurs during action potentials. When the action potentials are linked to the pacesetter potential, coordinated gastric peristaltic waves are propagated from the corpus through the antrum to the pylorus (Figure 6.2). Thus, normal gastric contractility and normal gastric emptying rates are produced by the myoelectrical events of the stomach pacesetter and action potentials.

The origin of the pacesetter potentials remains an area of active investigation. The site of the intrinsic rhythmicity of the stomach appears to be located in the interstitial cells of Cajal. These are specialized cells with properties of neural and smooth muscle elements. The cells are laid out in a meshwork between the longitudinal and circular muscle layers of the stomach and are in close proximity to the myenteric neurones.

Abnormalities of the electrical and contractile elements described above may develop in regions of the stomach ranging from the fundus to the body to the antrum and duodenum (Figure 6.3). For example, fundic relaxation in response to ingestion of food may be either excessive or insufficient and result in abnormal fundic relaxation, which is associated with bloating. Antral hypomotility may result from abnormal gastric pacesetter activity or abnormal action-potential activity, both of which may disrupt normal postprandial contractions and emptying rates.

Gastroparesis, or delayed gastric emptying, is the most extreme form of gastric neuromuscular dysfunction. In this situation, a standard meal is

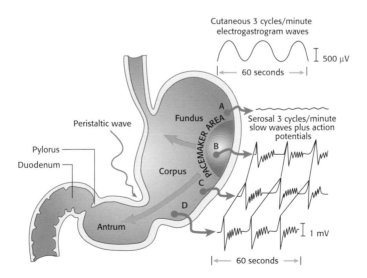

Figure 6.2 Slow waves or pacesetter potentials arise from the pacemaker area. Action potentials and pacesetter potentials are linked to corpus and antral circular muscle contraction, and form the electrical basis of the antral peristaltic wave. A, B, C and D are serosal electrodes.

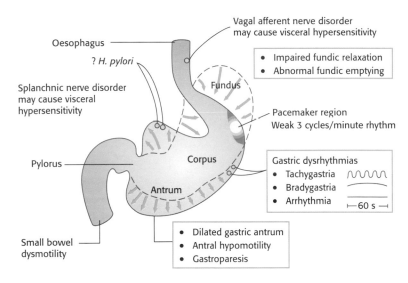

Figure 6.3 Spectrum of neuromuscular dysfunction in dyspepsia. Reproduced with permission from Koch and Stern. *Semin Gastrointest Dis* 1996;4:185–95.

not emptied within the range of normal emptying times. In patients with functional dyspepsia defined by vague epigastric discomfort, the incidence of gastroparesis ranges from 20 to 50%. In many patients, viral gastro-enteritis or flu-like illness precedes the gastroparesis. Causes of the condition are summarized in Table 6.1.

Gastric dysrhythmias are often found in patients with delayed gastric emptying. They are described as tachygastrias, in which abnormal electrical frequencies range from 3.75 to 10.0 cpm, or bradygastrias, in which abnormal frequencies range from 1.0 to 2.5 cpm (Figure 6.3).

Gastric dysrhythmias have been recorded in adults and children with dyspepsia symptoms and normal gastric emptying. A recent study showed that 60% of patients with dysmotility-like dyspepsia have gastric dysrhythmias. They may be one of the pathophysiological mechanisms associated with postprandial symptoms. The association is supported by the finding that resolution of gastric dysrhythmias and establishment of a normal 3-cpm gastric electrical rhythm is associated with symptom improvement during treatment with domperidone or cisapride.

Disordered intragastric distribution of meals. Patients with dyspepsia have decreased fundal compliance and ingested meals are moved into

TABLE 6.1

Causes of gastroparesis*

Mechanical obstruction

- Pylorus
- Duodenum
- Small intestine

Postgastric surgery

- Vagotomy
- Antrectomy
- Roux-en-Y
- Fundoplication

Metabolic/endocrine disorders

- Diabetes mellitus
- Hypothyroidism
- Hyperthyroidism
- Adrenal insufficiency

Medications

- Anticholinergic agents
- Narcotics
- L-dopa
- Progesterone
- Oestrogen
- Calcium-channel blockers

Mesenteric ischaemia

Psychogenic disorders

- Anorexia nervosa
- Bulimia

Smooth-muscle disorders

- Hollow-viscus myopathy
- Scleroderma
- Muscular dystrophy

Neuropathic disorders

- Hollow-viscus neuropathy
- Parkinson's disease
- Paraneoplastic syndrome
- Shy-Drager syndrome

Postviral gastroparesis

Idiopathic disorders

- Idiopathic gastroparesis with gastric dysrhythmia

*Modified from Koch 1997

the antrum sooner after the meal compared with controls. The altered intragastric movement of food may also evoke dyspepsia symptoms.

Antral dilatation. Ultrasound studies have shown that the antrum is dilated in patients with functional dysmotility-type dyspepsia. The extent of dilatation correlates with the intensity of bloating symptoms.

Gastric hypersensitivity. Patients with dyspepsia experience discomfort and pain at significantly lower volumes of intragastric balloon distension compared with healthy control subjects. Compliance measures of the fundus, however, are similar in both groups. These findings infer that the dyspeptic patient may have a 'visceral hypersensitivity' to distension of the stomach. In addition, the fundus does not relax normally in response to duodenal distension in functional dyspepsia, a finding that suggests duodenogastric reflexes are abnormal.

H. pylori. The role of *H. pylori* as a causative agent in dysmotility-like dyspepsia remains controversial. Recent studies show that eradication therapy in patients with dyspepsia symptoms and *H. pylori* infection results in only a small percentage of patients reporting symptom improvement (20% or less).

Hormones. Dyspepsia symptoms are often worse premenstrually. Neuromuscular function of the stomach may be affected by the levels of hormones related to the menstrual cycle. Oestrogen and progesterone evoke nausea and gastric dysrhythmias in healthy women. The release of hormones may further worsen subtle neuromuscular abnormalities of the stomach and create additional symptoms at these times.

Stress. Acute and chronic physical or psychological stresses or history of abuse may also affect the autonomic nervous system, alter neural hormonal secretions and ultimately affect gastric neuromuscular activities. Studies have shown that patients with chronic dyspepsia do not have obvious psychological profiles or psychiatric disorders. However, anxiety and somatization are present in patients with dysmotility-type chronic dyspepsia.

Clinical presentation

Clinicians should focus on the predominant symptom. If this is epigastric pain, then ulcer-like dyspepsia is the most appropriate diagnosis. If the range of symptoms includes mainly postprandial bloating, fullness, early satiety, nausea and vomiting, a diagnosis of dysmotility-like dyspepsia is better. Symptoms of dysmotility-like dyspepsia may be present during the fasted states, but they usually increase postprandially. Patients often feel poorly after they eat and so modify their diet to minimize symptoms. For the diagnosis of functional dyspepsia, standard diagnostic tests should be normal and symptoms must be present for 3 months or more.

Diagnosis

The diagnosis of ulcer-like or dysmotility-like functional dyspepsia requires that standard diseases and disorders are excluded. As mentioned previously, the symptoms of dyspepsia are non-specific and therefore GORD, peptic ulcer disease, irritable bowel syndrome, and biliary and pancreatic diseases must be excluded.

Acid peptic diseases, such as GORD, gastric or duodenal ulcer disease, often have some element of a 'burning' sensation in the epigastrium. If the sensation rises into the substernal area, GORD may be diagnosed. Some patients with GORD also have gastric motility disorders, an overlap syndrome that defines dysmotility-like dyspepsia and GORD symptoms.

Organic disease often occurs in patients with chronic dyspepsia. In a recent study:

- 24% of patients had GORD
- 21% had gastritis or duodenitis
- 20% had peptic ulcer disease
- 2% had gastrointestinal cancer.

Thus, 67% of patients had specific and accepted diagnoses after investigation, even though they had presented with non-specific dyspeptic symptoms.

Biliary and pancreatic disease. Chronic cholecystitis may also present with non-specific symptoms of postprandial discomfort, bloating and nausea. Pain or discomfort due to biliary diseases is often exacerbated by meals. In a questionnaire study, it was found that, of the patients with 'dyspepsia':

- 30% had irritable bowel syndrome
- 29% had GORD
- 25% had a combination of irritable bowel syndrome and gastro-oesophageal reflux.

Only 6% had gallstones. It is unclear whether or not the gallstones were related to the predominant symptoms reported by the patient.

It may be difficult to determine the relevance of gallstones to a pain syndrome described by an individual patient. If the gall bladder wall is thickened or oedematous on ultrasound examination, the evidence suggests chronic inflammation. A gall bladder-emptying study may also indicate disordered contractile function of the gall bladder, a finding associated with chronic cholecystitis.

Chronic pancreatitis is usually accompanied by a moderate-to-severe pain in the epigastrium that radiates into the back. In the presence of increased lipase or amylase, this is not a difficult diagnosis to confirm. More difficult are diagnoses of biliary stenosis or sphincter of Oddi spasm, which may also present with right upper quadrant or with gastric post-prandial discomfort.

Small bowel disorders and chronic mesenteric ischaemia. In the postprandial period, mesenteric blood flow increases and the small intestine enters a postprandial contractile phase. The small bowel may contribute to postprandial symptoms if strictures, adhesions or narrowings create a bowel obstruction. Small bowel lesions can be subtle and difficult to detect.

Chronic mesenteric ischaemia may be due to atherosclerotic disease, intimal hyperplasia or aneurysmal damage to two of the three major abdominal vessels. The ischaemic discomfort is usually increased in the postprandial period, but it may be a mild, non-descript pain. Chronic mesenteric ischaemia should be considered in the differential diagnosis of dysmotility-like dyspepsia. Symptoms and gastroparesis resolve with vascular bypass surgery.

Standard tests

The approach for an uninvestigated dyspepsia patient is described in Chapter 1. If dyspepsia symptoms have not responded to initial empirical therapy or if there are alarm symptoms, the following clinical approach is suggested to investigate the symptoms.

First, have empirical treatments of GORD, peptic ulcer disease or a neuromuscular abnormality of the stomach been carried out? This usually involves 3–6 weeks of an appropriate drug, such as an H_2-receptor antagonist, proton-pump inhibitor or a promotility agent. Such an approach assumes that there are no alarm features.

If the patient does not respond or if alarm symptoms are present, a UGI series, barium meal or a UGI endoscopy is the appropriate first step in evaluation. The UGI series will exclude:

- gross reflux of gastric content into the oesophagus
- large ulcers
- gross obstruction at the antrum, pylorus or duodenum.

Upper gastrointestinal endoscopy will detect these findings and more subtle signs of oesophagitis, gastritis or duodenitis. Antral biopsies can also be obtained to determine whether or not *H. pylori* infection is present.

If studies of the oesophagus, stomach and duodenum are normal, an ultrasound examination of the gall bladder should be performed. This will exclude cholelithiasis and evidence of gall-bladder or peri gall-bladder inflammation. Dilatation of the common bile duct or cystic duct can also be established. Although bowel gas frequently obscures the view, ultrasound may also identify the pancreas and rule out significant pancreatic inflammation, pseudocysts or other retroperitoneal abnormalities that might be associated with the dyspepsia symptoms.

Thus, if imaging plus routine blood studies fail to identify a common or uncommon structural, biochemical or infectious cause of the symptoms, a diagnosis of functional dyspepsia can be made.

Unfortunately, investigation of the patient with dysmotility-like dyspepsia frequently ends after a normal endoscopy and/or normal ultrasound are obtained. A diagnostic work-up should continue beyond endoscopy and should address gastric neuromuscular function. A number of non-invasive and invasive tests of gastric motility are available and each test measures a different aspect of gastric neuromuscular activity (Table 6.2).

Non-invasive tests for gastric neuromuscular abnormalities. Diagnostic methods to measure aspects of gastric motility vary in the level of radiation to which the patient is exposed, invasiveness and time required to perform the test.

Gastric emptying tests are usually performed in nuclear medicine departments. The test food is labelled with an isotope and the isotope is identified within the stomach with a gamma camera. The number of counts from the region of interest is calculated over time and expressed as a percentage of the meal emptied or retained. A gastric-emptying curve is

TABLE 6.2

Gastric motility tests

Test	Result
Solid/liquid gastric emptying (nuclear medicine)	Global stomach function
Electrogastrography	Gastric dysrhythmia
Gastric ultrasound	Antral dilatation
Gastric barostatography	Relaxation/contraction of fundus
Gastroduodenal manometry	Intraluminal pressures in antrum, duodenum, small bowel

constructed that reflects the rate of gastric emptying of the test meal. The test exposes the patient to the approximate equivalent of one or two abdominal radiograph films. Although gastroparesis is diagnosed by this test, the underlying mechanism is not determined. Intragastric distribution of food can also be assessed.

Electrogastrography is a non-invasive technique for recording gastric electrical activity. Electrodes are placed on the abdominal surface in the epigastrium, and the electrogastrogram (EGG) reflects the myoelectrical rhythms of the stomach, much like an ECG reflects electrical rhythms of the heart. The normal gastric myoelectrical rhythm is 3 cpm (range 2.5–3.75 cpm) and the rhythm detected by the EGG is similar to the pacesetter potential frequencies recorded by serosal or mucosal electrodes. Abnormal rhythms include bradygastrias (flatline or 1.0–2.5 cpm), tachygastrias and tachyarrhythmias (3.75–10.0 cpm). Duodenal respiratory frequency rates range from 10 to 15 cpm. Gastric dysrhythmias have been detected in a variety of clinical and research situations in which nausea is a prominent symptom, including dysmotility-like dyspepsia.

Gastric ultrasound. The antral diameter is measured at several time points after ingestion of standard liquid meals. The rate of gastric emptying is estimated from changes in the antral diameter.

Gastric barostatography. A gastric barostat is a balloon device, mounted on catheters, which is passed into the stomach via the mouth. The balloon is inflated to a set basal pressure. Subsequent changes in fundic pressure or tone are reflected by changes in the balloon volume as air is either expelled from the balloon or infused into the balloon to maintain the constant basal pressure.

Gastroduodenal manometry. Perfused catheters or solid-phase pressure transducers mounted on flexible catheters are positioned fluoroscopically in the gastric antrum and duodenum to measure intraluminal pressures. Intraluminal pressure changes are registered only if the stomach or duodenal muscle wall contracts to obliterate the lumen. Such devices fail to measure contractions that do not occlude the lumen. Gastroduodenal manometry tests are invasive and require 10–30 seconds of fluoroscopy time to determine the tube's position.

Non-invasive gastric neuromuscular evaluation. The results of EGG and gastric-emptying tests can be divided into four diagnostic categories (Figure 6.4). These reflect different pathophysiological findings that may affect the patient's diagnosis and management.

Gastric dysrhythmia and gastroparesis. These findings provide evidence of a diffuse electrical and contractile abnormality of the stomach. The causes of gastroparesis must be reviewed (see Table 6.1).

High-amplitude, normal 3-cpm EGG pattern and gastroparesis are suggestive of gastric-outlet or small-bowel obstruction.

Gastric dysrhythmia and normal gastric emptying. Gastric dysrhythmia indicates abnormal electrical activity, but the abnormality is not severe enough to affect gastric emptying. The dysrhythmia may have a role in the generation of the dysmotility-like dyspepsia symptoms. Correction of the gastric dysrhythmia with a prokinetic drug, such as cisapride or domperidone, is associated with improvement in symptoms.

Normal 3-cpm EGG pattern and normal gastric emptying. These patients have no evidence of contractile or electrical abnormalities of the stomach. Other disorders should be investigated or re-investigated as a potential cause of symptoms. For example, delayed gall-bladder emptying may be a cause of postprandial symptoms. If occult GORD was not excluded, then a 24-hour oesophageal pH test should be considered. Diseases or disorders of the central nervous system must also be excluded in patients with recurrent nausea and vomiting, and normal gastric emptying and EGG.

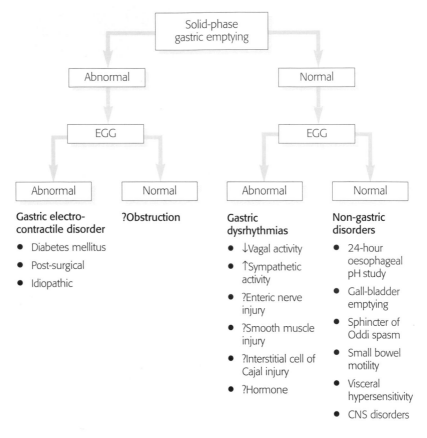

Figure 6.4 In dyspepsia patients, non-invasive physiological testing for gastric electrical and contractile dysfunction can determine four categories of neuromuscular dysfunction.

There may be other subtle disorders of gastric and duodenal neuro-muscular dysfunction (e.g. pylorospasm or visceral hypersensitivity). Pylorospasm may or may not result in gastroparesis. Visceral hypersensitivity is associated with increased pain on balloon distension of the fundus. Diagnosis of these abnormalities usually requires special invasive, diagnostic procedures with manometric catheters or a barostat.

Treatment

With a specific diagnosis, more directed or aggressive therapy can be provided. For example, if the 24-hour oesophageal pH study shows that frequent acid-reflux episodes are associated with symptoms, either a more aggressive approach to acid suppression can be initiated or prokinetic therapy started. If the major pathological finding is delayed gall-bladder emptying and if other possibilities have been excluded, cholecystectomy may relieve symptoms. Similarly, once a diagnosis is made on the basis of gastric emptying and dysrhythmia, several different therapeutic options are available.

Drug therapy. Patients with gastroparesis and gastric dysrhythmia have severe gastric neuromuscular dysfunction and may require aggressive treatment with gastric prokinetic or combination therapy. Patients should be given a realistic expectation of the benefits that they should experience with this kind of treatment.

Very few drugs are available currently to treat functional dyspepsia (Table 6.3). If the symptoms are ulcer-like, more aggressive acid-suppressant therapy may be tried. For dysmotility-like dyspepsia symptoms: metoclopramide, 10–20 mg, four times a day; cisapride, 10–20 mg, four times a day; or domperidone, 10–20 mg, four times a day, may be given. Prokinetic drugs generally reduce functional dyspepsia symptoms more effectively than H_2-receptor antagonists or placebo. The macrolide antibiotic erythromycin stimulates antral contractility and improves the gastric emptying rate.

Combination therapy has not been well studied; it should probably be given in consultation with a gastroenterologist because of the risk of potentially adverse interactions. For example, erythromycin is contraindicated in patients receiving cisapride because of the potential for ventricular dysrhythmia. Drug studies that focus on one or two predominant dyspepsia symptoms, such as bloating or nausea, have not been performed, thus drugs should be tried empirically.

Metoclopramide is a D_2-receptor antagonist in the brain and stomach. It also stimulates acetylcholine release from the myenteric neurones and has some $5\text{-}HT_3$ receptor antagonist activity. Metoclopramide is an anti-emetic and gastric prokinetic drug.

Side-effects. Metoclopramide is associated with central nervous system side-effects. These include:
- depression
- confusion

TABLE 6.3

Treatment of functional dyspepsia

Agent	Rationale
Ulcer-like dyspepsia	
H_2-receptor antagonist	● Acid sensitivity
Proton-pump inhibitor	● Acid sensitivity
Dysmotility-like dyspepsia	
Cisapride	● Acetylcholine deficit
Metoclopramide	● ?Dopamine excess ● ?Acetylcholine deficit
Domperidone	● ?Dopamine excess
Fedotozine (not available in the UK/USA)	● ?Opiate pathway dysfunction

- mental-status changes
- tardive dyskinesia.

Overall, 20–30% of patients taking metoclopramide will experience one or more side-effects that increase with higher doses.

Cisapride releases acetylcholine from the myenteric plexus, stimulating contractions in the small bowel and colon as well as the stomach. This can result in abdominal cramps and diarrhoea. Cisapride also competes with other prescription drugs for the liver enzyme cytochrome P_{450} 3A4. As a result, increased blood levels of cisapride may occur when it is prescribed with:

- macrolide antibiotics
- antifungal agents
- antidepressants, such as paroxetine and nefazodone
- protease inhibitors.

High blood levels of cisapride may result, together with an increased incidence of ventricular dysrhythmia.

Domperidone is associated with increases in prolactin levels and a 5–10% incidence of prolactin-related side-effects, such as breast tenderness.

Effect	Mechanism
• Acid suppression	• H$_2$-receptor blockade
• Acid suppression	• H$^+$/K$^+$ ATPase inhibitor
• Increased gastric contractions • Decreased gastric dysrhythmia	• Increased acetylcholine release by 5-HT$_4$ agonist
• Increased gastric contractions	• Dopamine antagonist (central and peripheral) • Increased acetylcholine release
• Increased gastric contractions • Decreased gastric dysrhythmia	• Dopamine antagonist (peripheral)
• ?Decreased visceral sensitivity	• Kappa agonist

Erythromycin is associated with abdominal cramps, nausea and vomiting, and is not tolerated by many patients with functional dyspepsia.

Dietary therapy. Patients may find some benefit in modifying their diet. In the presence of gastric electrical and contractile abnormalities, the volume of food ingested should be reduced so that six smaller meals are consumed during the day, rather than three main meals. The patient should be encouraged to snack frequently, so that larger volumes of liquid or solid foods do not stimulate dyspeptic symptoms. A three-step diet for patients with nausea and vomiting has been suggested (Table 6.4).

In patients who cannot tolerate oral intake, are losing weight and under-nourished, a gastrostomy tube for venting to prevent nausea and a jejunostomy for enteral feeding to maintain nutritional intake and weight stability may be necessary.

Non-drug therapies. Several non-drug therapies are in development. They include acustimulation or acupuncture to relieve chronic nausea. For severe, drug-refractory nausea and vomiting due to gastroparesis, gastric

TABLE 6.4

A three-step diet for patients with nausea and vomiting*

Symptoms	Recommended foods

Severe	• Liquids such as:
	  – commercial sports drinks with glucose, salt and potassium
	  – bouillon
	• Daily vitamin supplement

Less severe	• Foods such as:
	  – soups with noodles or rice
	  – crackers
	  – some candies/confectionery
	• Daily vitamin supplement

Relatively mild	• Solid foods such as:
	  – noodles
	  – rice
	  – potatoes
	  – white meat
	• Daily vitamin supplement

*Modified from Koch 1995

pacemaking devices have reduced symptoms, and improved gastric dysrhythmia and gastric-emptying rates in small numbers of selected patients. These exciting non-drug therapies appear promising and clinical research will indicate the settings in which these therapeutic modalities are appropriate.

CHAPTER 7

Future trends

Towards safer NSAID therapy

NSAIDs are invaluable in the management of inflammatory arthritis, but are unfortunately associated with a high risk of gastroduodenal mucosal damage. Their efficacy depends largely on inhibition of the enzyme cyclo-oxygenase (COX), which is essential for the production of inflammatory prostaglandins. All NSAIDs available at the time of press inhibit, to a variable degree, the COX responsible for the production of both physiological prostaglandins (COX-1) and the pathological prostaglandins (COX-2). The physiological prostaglandins are important for maintaining the integrity of the gastroduodenal mucosa.

Theoretically, a drug that does not inhibit COX-1, but remains effective against COX-2, should have the advantage of combining anti-inflammatory activity with a lower gastroduodenal mucosal toxicity. Meloxicam has been promoted as a relatively selective COX-2 inhibitor, but it is not entirely without gastrointestinal side-effects. More highly selective COX-2 inhibitor drugs have been introduced recently but their efficacy and toxicity will need to be assessed.

An alternative approach to safer NSAID therapy is to link the anti-inflammatory drug to a nitric oxide-donating agent. Local nitric-oxide production appears to protect the gastroduodenal mucosa by its vasodilatory effect, but results of human studies are not yet available.

Towards more cost-effective control of *H. pylori*

The incidence of *H. pylori* infection and associated diseases has declined in industrialized countries during the past 30 years, largely due to improved hygiene and living standards. It is reasonable to predict that, as similar changes take place in the developing world, the same trend will also be seen in these countries. Nevertheless, a more effective means of controlling and eradicating the infection than is currently available would be a major contribution to world health.

Future antibiotics. The genomic sequence of *H. pylori* is now known and this has provided the means of identifying which of its genes are essential for viability. The products of such genes include those necessary for the synthesis of nucleic acids and proteins, particularly those involved in maintaining the integrity of cell membranes. Recombinant gene technology will facilitate the production of these proteins for use in studies that will, in turn, enable highly specific 'antibiotic' drugs to be developed.

Vaccination. Although it may prove possible to eradicate *H. pylori* in the future with target-specific drugs, worldwide control of the infection is likely to depend on the development of a vaccine. In most circumstances, a vaccine is given prophylactically to uninfected people to produce antibodies that prevent clinical infection on subsequent contact with the organism. This may well prove possible in respect of *H. pylori*. However, universal preventive vaccination may not be cost-effective, even in the developed world.

An alternative is 'therapeutic immunization', which involves vaccinating those already infected to boost the host response to a level that leads to eradication. Experiments in mice and ferrets have been successful, but it will be several years before a product is available commercially. Nevertheless, when available, immunization of serologically screened subjects with this type of vaccine might be more feasible and cost-effective than universal prophylactic vaccination or antibiotic therapy.

Towards improved diagnosis and treatment of GORD

Increasingly, proton-pump inhibitors will become the basic treatment for typical heartburn due to GORD. Patients with GORD and symptoms of gastric dysmotility (GORD plus) will be recognized as a distinct patient subgroup and given combination therapy with proton-pump inhibitors and prokinetic agents. Also, atypical symptoms of GORD will be better understood, properly diagnosed and effectively treated. These developments will have a significant impact on the diagnosis and treatment of disorders such as asthma, aspiration pneumonia, chronic cough and hoarseness.

As the cost of endoscopy decreases in the USA, a greater number of patients with chronic heartburn symptoms will undergo this procedure to establish the presence or absence of Barrett's epithelium. However, tests to identify at-risk patients are needed to ensure endoscopies are only performed on appropriate patient populations. This may lead to a decreasing incidence of oesophageal cancer.

Continually improving laparoscopic surgical techniques will make surgery an option for more patients with drug-refractory heartburn or atypical symptoms of GORD. Appropriate pre-operative evaluation of oesophageal and gastric motility will be an increasingly important consideration for these patients to ensure optimal surgical outcome.

Future investigations into the pathophysiology of GORD may reveal new mechanisms that will lead to the development of new treatments. Improved therapy based on the known mechanisms of GORD, such as transient lower oesophageal sphincter relaxations, will also become a reality. The relevance of other agents injurious to the oesophageal mucosa, such as bile acids, pancreatic juices and *H. pylori*, will also be clarified further.

Towards improved diagnosis and treatment of functional dyspepsia

At present, functional dyspepsia is a rather ill-defined clinical area. Our understanding of the pathophysiology and treatment of dyspepsia should improve greatly in the future, thus clarifying the meaning of the term. 'Functional dyspepsia' has little meaning for patients and is poorly defined in the minds of most physicians. Indeed, it will probably be abandoned altogether with time. In the future, it is possible that the pathophysiological mechanisms involved in the condition will be shown not to be functional, but in fact neuromuscular and/or hormonal.

The pathophysiological mechanisms of nausea and bloating will be clearly defined in coming years allowing the development of new and more specific medical and non-medical treatments. For example, gastric pacemaker therapy may become a reality for severe gastroparesis. Acustimulation, acupuncture and herbal medicines may also be used more often to treat these symptoms in mild to moderately severe gastric neuromuscular disorders.

Understanding of the parasympathetic and sympathetic afferent nervous system pathways that carry information from peripheral organs in the gastrointestinal system to the central nervous system, where inflammation or neuromuscular/hormonal dysfunction is perceived as noxious sensations, such as nausea, fullness and bloating, will be important. New classes of treatment will be developed to modulate such afferent neural traffic.

Key references

GENERAL

British Society of Gastroenterology Dyspepsia Management Guidelines, September 1996.

Jones C. *Practical Approach to Dyspepsia*. Oxford: The Medicine Group, 1989.

Lydeard S, Jones R. Factors affecting the decision to consult with dyspepsia: a comparison of consulters with non-consulters. *J R Coll Gen Pract* 1989;39:495–8.

McColl KEL. Pathophysiology of duodenal ulcer disease. *Eur J Gastroenterol* 1997;9(Suppl 1):S9–12.

Sonnenberg A, Townsend WF. Costs of duodenal ulcer therapy with antibiotics. *Arch Intern Med* 1995;155:922–8.

GASTRO-OESOPHAGEAL REFLUX DISEASE

Barlow AB, DeMeester TR, Ball CS *et al.* The significance of the gastric secretory state in gastroesophageal reflux disease. *Arch Surg* 1989;124:937–40.

Bell NJV, Hunt RH. Role of gastric acid suppression in the treatment of gastroesophageal reflux disease. *Gut* 1991;33:1118–24.

Brossard E, Monnier JB, Ollyo JB *et al.* Serious complications – stenosis, ulcer and Barrett's epithelium – develop in 21.6% of adults with erosive reflux esophagitis. *Gastroenterology* 1992; 100:A36.

Brzana RJ, Koch KL. Intractable nausea presenting as gastroesophageal reflux disease. *Ann Intern Med* 1997;126: 704–7.

Dakkat M, Jones BP, Scott MGB *et al.* Comparing the efficacy of cisapride and ranitidine in esophagitis: a double-blind, parallel group study in general practice. *Br J Clin Pract* 1994;48:10–14.

El-Searg HB, Sonnenberg A. Comorbid occurrence of laryngeal or pulmonary disease with esophagitis in United States' military veterans. *Gastroenterology* 1997;113:755–60.

Fennerti MB, Sampliner RE, Garewell HS. Review: Barrett's oesophagus – cancer risk, biology and therapeutic management. *Aliment Pharmacol Ther* 1993;7:339–45.

Hinder RA, Filipi CJ, Wetschler G *et al.* Laparoscopic Nissen fundoplication is an effective treatment for gastroesophageal reflux disease. *Ann Surg* 1994;220:472–83.

Johnson LF, DeMeester TR. Twenty-four hour pH monitoring of the distal esophagus. *Am J Gastroenterol* 1974;62:325–32.

Katz PO. Pathogenesis and management of gastroesophageal reflux disease. *J Clin Gastroenterol* 1991;113:S6–15.

Klinkenberg-Knoll EC, Festen HPM, Jansen JBMJ *et al.* Long-term treatment with omeprazole for refractory reflux esophagitis: efficacy and safety. *Ann Intern Med* 1994;121:161–7.

Lock G, Holsteg A, Lang B *et al*. Gastrointestinal manifestations of progressive systemic sclerosis. *Am J Gastroenterol* 1997;92:763–71.

McCallum RW, Berkowitz DM, Lerner E. Gastric emptying in patients with gastroesophageal reflux. *Gastroenterology* 1981;80:285–91.

Mittal K, McCallum RW. Characteristics and frequency of transient relaxations of the lower oesophageal sphincter on patients with reflux esophagitis. *Gastroenterology* 1988;95:593 9.

Orlando RC. Reflux esophagitis. In: T Yamada, ed. *Textbook of Gastroenterology*. Philadelphia: JB Lippincott, 1995:1318–46.

Schnatz PF, Castell JA, Castell DO. Pulmonary symptoms associated with gastroesophageal reflux: use of ambulatory pH monitoring to diagnose and to direct therapy. *Am J Gastroenterol* 1996;91:1715–18.

Viaezi MF, Richter JE. Role of acid and duodenogastroesophageal reflux in gastroesophageal reflux disease. *Gastroenterology* 1996;111:1192–9.

Winder GJ, Morgan TM, Cooper JB *et al*. Ambulatory 24 hour oesophageal monitoring: reproducibility and variability of pH parameters. *Dig Dis Sci* 1988;33:1127–30.

H. PYLORI

Banatvala N, Mayo K, Megraud F *et al*. The cohort effect and *Helicobacter pylori*. *J Infect Dis* 1993;168:219–21.

Calam J. *Clinician's Guide to* Helicobacter pylori. London: Chapman & Hall, 1996.

Dixon MF. *Helicobacter pylori* and peptic ulceration: histopathological aspects. *J Gastroenterol Hepatol* 1991;6:125–30.

The European *Helicobacter Pylori* Study Group. The Maastricht Consensus Report. *Gut* 1997;41:8–13.

Forman D, Newell DG, Fullerton F *et al*. Association between infection with *Helicobacter pylori* and risk of gastric cancer; evidence from a prospective investigation. *BMJ* 1991;302:1302–5.

Fox JG. Postulated transmission of *H. pylori*. *Aliment Pharmacol Ther* 1995; 9(Suppl 2):93–103.

Graham DY, Hepps KS, Raminez FC *et al*. Treatment of *Helicobacter pylori* reduces the rate of re-bleeding in peptic ulcer disease. *Scand J Gastroenterol* 1993;28:939–42.

Jaspersen D. Helicobacter eradication: the best long term prophylaxis for ulcer bleeding recurrence? *Endoscopy* 1995;27:622–5.

Labenze J, Borch G. Role of *Helicobacter pylori* eradication in the prevention of peptic ulcer bleeding relapse. *Digestion* 1994;55:19–23.

Marshall BJ, Goodwin CS, Warren JR *et al*. Prospective double-blind trial of duodenal ulcer relapse after eradication of *Campylobacter pylori*. *Lancet* 1988;2:1437–42.

Marshall BJ. The 1995 Albert Lasker Medical Research Award. *Helicobacter pylori*. The etiologic agent for peptic ulcer. *JAMA* 1995;274:1064–6.

Misiewicz JT. Management of *Helicobacter pylori*-related disorders. *Eur J Gastroenterol Hepatol* 1997;9(Suppl 1):S17–21.

Nomara A, Stemmermann GV, Chyou PH *et al. Helicobacter pylori* and gastric carcinoma among Japanese Americans in Hawaii. *N Engl J Med* 1991;325:1132–6.

Northfield TC, Mendall M, Coggin PM, eds. *Helicobacter pylori infection.* Dordrecht: Kluwer, 1993.

Parson J, Friedman GD, Vandersteen DP *et al. Helicobacter pylori* infection and the risk of gastric carcinoma. *N Engl J Med* 1991;325:1127–31.

Primary Care Society for *Gastroenterology.* Decision points for the management of *H. pylori* in primary care, March 1997.

Rokkas T, Karameris A, Maurogeorgis A *et al.* Eradication of *Helicobacter pylori* reduces the possibility of re-bleeding in peptic ulcer disease. *Gastrointest Endosc* 1994;41:1–4.

PEPTIC ULCER

Baron JH. Peptic ulcer: a problem almost solved. *J R Coll Physicians Lond* 1997;31:512–20.

Calam J. *Clinician's Guide to* Helicobacter Pylori. London: Chapman and Hall, 1996:54.

Gear MWL. The place of surgery in the management of peptic ulcer. A comparison with modern drug therapy. In: Lancaster Smith MJ, ed. *Peptic Ulcer.* London: Update Siebert, 1986.

Griffen MR, Piper JM, Daugherty JR *et al.* Non-steroidal anti-inflammatory drug use and increased risk for peptic ulcer disease in elderly persons. *Ann Intern Med* 1991;114:257–63.

Kurata JH. Ulcer epidemiology: an overview and proposed research framework. *Gastroenterology* 1989;96:569–80.

Kurata JH, Honda GD, Frankl H. The incidence of duodenal and gastric ulcers in a large health maintenance organization. *Am J Public Health* 1985;75:625–9.

Sonnenberg A, Townsend WF. Costs of duodenal ulcer therapy with antibiotics. *Arch Intern Med* 1995;155:922–8.

Sussen M. Period effects, generation effects and age effects in peptic ulcer mortality. *J Chronic Dis* 1982;35:29–40.

CARCINOMA OF THE OESOPHAGUS AND STOMACH

Kuipers EJ. Review: Exploring the link between *Helicobacter pylori* and gastric cancer. *Aliment Pharmacol Ther* 1999;13(Suppl 1):3–11.

FUNCTIONAL DYSPEPSIA

Coffin B, Aspiroz F, Guarner F *et al.* Selective gastric hypersensitivity and reflex hyporeactivity in functional dyspepsia. *Gastroenterology* 1994;107:1345–51.

Cucchiara S, Minella R, Riezzo G *et al.* Reversal of gastric electrical dysrhythmias by cisapride in children with functional dyspepsia: report of three cases. *Dig Dis Sci* 1992;37:1136–40.

Dobrilla G, Comberlato M, Steele A *et al.* Drug treatment of functional dyspepsia: meta analysis of randomized controlled clinical trials. *J Clin Gastroenterol* 1989;11:169–77.

Koch KL. Approach to the patient with nausea and vomiting. In: Yamada T, ed. *Textbook of Gastroenterology*. Philadelphia: JB Lippincott, 1995: 731–49.

Koch KL. The stomach. In: Schuster MM, ed. *Atlas of Gastrointestinal Motility in Health and Disease*. Baltimore: Williams & Wilkins, 1993:158–76.

Koch KL. Dyspepsia of unknown origin: pathophysiology, diagnosis and treatment. *Dig Dis* 1997;15:316–29.

Koch KL, Stern RM. Functional disorders of the stomach. *Semin Gastrointest Dis* 1996;4:185–95.

Koch KL, Stern RM. Electrogastrography. In: Kumar D, Wingate D, eds. *Illustrated Guide to Gastrointestinal Motility*. London: Churchill Livingstone, 1993:290–307.

Liberski SM, Koch KL, Atnip RG *et al*. Ischemic gastroparesis: resolution of nausea, vomiting and gastroparesis after mesenteric artery revascularization. *Gastroenterology* 1990;99:252–7.

Lin HC, Hasler WL. Disorders of gastric emptying. In: T Yamada, ed. *Textbook of Gastroenterology*. Philadelphia: JB Lippincott, 1995:1318–46.

McCallum RW, Chen JDZ, Lin Z *et al*. Gastric pacing improves emptying and symptoms in patients with gastroparesis. *Gastroenterology* 1998;114:456–61.

Misiewicz JJ. Dyspepsia. In: Sleisenger J, Fordtran XX, eds. *Gastrointestinal Disease: Pathophysiology, Diagnosis, Management*. Philadelphia: Saunders, 1993:572–9.

Rothstein RD, Alavai A, Reynolds JC. Electrogastrography in patients with gastroparesis and effect of long-term cisapride. *Dig Dis Sci* 1993;38:1518–24.

Talley MJ, Colin-Jones D, Koch KL *et al*. Functional dyspepsia: a classification with guidelines for diagnosis and management. *Gastroenterol Int* 1991;4:145–60.

Troncon LEA, Bennett RJM, Ahluwalia NK *et al*. Abnormal intragastric distribution of food during gastric emptying in functional dyspepsia patients. *Gut* 1994;35:327–32.

Index

Other titles available in the *Fast Facts* series

To order, please contact:

Health Press Limited
Elizabeth House, Queen Street,
Abingdon, Oxford OX14 3JR, UK
Tel: +44 (0)1235 523233
Fax: +44 (0)1235 523238
Email: post@healthpress.co.uk

Or visit our website:
www.healthpress.co.uk

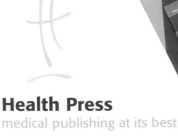

Health Press
medical publishing at its best

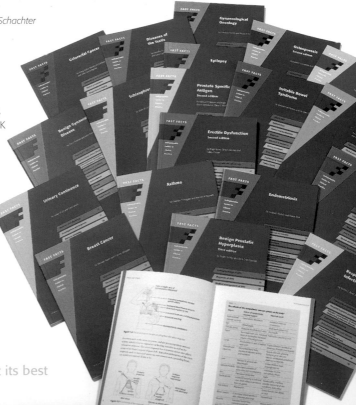